Handle with Care

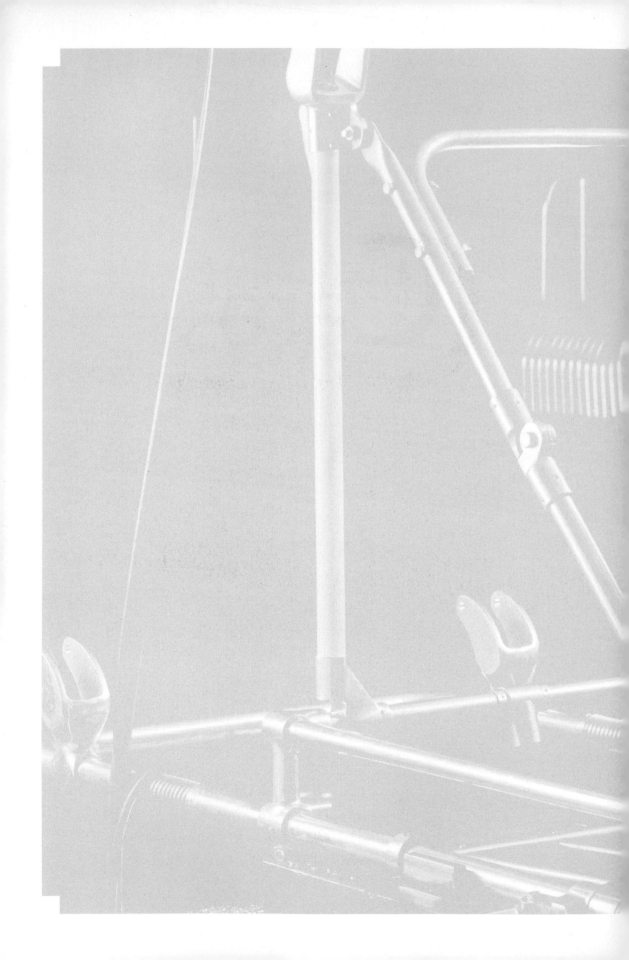

Handle with Care

The Ferno Story

Shaping Emergency Care
Around the World

Laura Pulfer

ORANGE *frazer* PRESS
Wilmington, Ohio

ISBN 978-1939710-314
Copyright©2015 Ferno-Washington, Inc.

Published for Ferno-Washington, Inc. by:
Orange Frazer Press
P.O. Box 214
Wilmington, OH 45177

Telephone: 937.382.3196 for price and shipping information.
Website: www.orangefrazer.com
Book and cover design: Alyson Rua and Orange Frazer Press

 Library of Congress Cataloging-in-Publication Data

Pulfer, Laura, 1946-
  Handle with care : the Ferno story, shaping emergency care around the world / Laura Pulfer.
    pages cm
  Includes index.
  ISBN 978-1-939710-31-4
  1. Ferno (Firm) 2. Medical supplies industry--United States. 3. Transport of sick and wounded--United States. 4. Emergency medical services--United States. I. Title.
  HD9994.U54F477 2015
  338.7'681761--dc23
                        2015022708

This book is dedicated to the Ferno Family, past and present. It's our *people*, from the Blue Room to manufacturing and logistics, from sales to finance, from customer service to after-sale service, to boardrooms around the world, who never forgot, and now continue to remember, that they work for the patients on Ferno stretchers and for the people who carry them. We thank them all for being part of the Ferno Family. The Ferno Way is a culture focused on three core attributes of integrity, excellence, and innovation. The Ferno Family's sixty years of incredible loyalty and fierce dedication, whose passion and purpose has served people around the world, are tangible qualities that we honor and respect. This story is your story. This company is your legacy.

Acknowledgments

We wish to thank everyone who helped to both shape and
capture the Ferno story for their invaluable contributions.

—*El & Elaine, Joe, Brian, and El-B Bourgraf*

Thank you to the many who contributed to the content of
the book. Those who gathered data from around the world, located
the unfindable from file drawers and boxes, openly shared their
keepsakes and memories, and worked tirelessly to capture Ferno's
story. It took a team of people to bring these stories to life.

—*Laura Pulfer*

Contents

Foreword

first met the Bourgraf Family at a swim meet. Elaine and El's son El-B was a high school American swimmer, and they were volunteering at the meet. At the time, I had never heard of Ferno Washington and I did not know that I was talking to the visionary who, with Dick Ferneau, had created the emergency patient handling industry. All I knew was that El had a big heart and cared about his fellow man. As I started representing Ferno and met Dick Ferneau, I learned that Dick also had a heart of gold.

Over the past thirty years, I have witnessed all the things El, Dick, and the Ferno Team did to enhance the lives of others. El has always been actively involved in numerous civic, charitable, and community organizations. Dick would quietly learn about families in his community who were struggling and then anonymously give them food, clothing, or money to address their needs. The Ferno Team follows these wonderful role models as they find ways to support each other and their communities in times of need.

When a family approached El and Dick about a specific need for their disabled child, Ferno developed a solution and then "conveniently" lost their invoice for the work because they knew the family did not have the financial resources to pay.

When you put together the Ferno Team's commitment to care for others, plus their knowledge that their own family members will someday need to use a Ferno product, you create the passion for the Ferno Team to develop the best possible products to save and protect you, me, and our families. This passion is part of Ferno's culture, which is why they have been so innovative and successful.

Ferno's innovation is a result of their ability to listen to the frontline players, the paramedics, and medical personnel to understand their needs and the needs of their patients. The collaborative process established by El then draws on the experience, vision, and passion of each member of the Ferno Team to bring out the best ideas to create life changing solutions.

El once told me that someday he will handle my body. Well, not yet, but I have already witnessed four generations of my family safely buckled onto a Ferno product to be transported to a hospital.

From a child's ride to a hospital on a Ferno Pedi-Pac® to a person's last ride at their funeral on a Ferno Church Truck, Ferno products protect us from cradle to grave. That's the scope of the industry that El and Dick created.

As you will learn from reading this book, the greatest achievement of El Bourgraf and Dick Ferneau is that they founded a business that saves, protects, and supports the value of human life and respects the dignity of the deceased—a business that embraces humanity.

I wish all the readers of this book well, but if you or a family member becomes sick or injured, I know you will have a safe ride on a Ferno product.

—*Bill Keating, Jr.*
Partner
Keating Muething & Klekamp PLL

Prologue

Just after September of 2001, a young man traveled from Ohio to New York City to replenish emergency equipment for the most celebrated fire department in the world, the FDNY. Pushing his face against a chain link fence at one of the firehouses, he peered at a stretcher in an enclosure behind a building. He recognized it. Maybe he had been the one to machine some of the castings or to assemble it. If not this stretcher, one just like it.

The cot was manufactured by his father's company. "It looked like it had gone through hell," Elroy Bourgraf Jr. said.

It had.

Restraint straps were melted, buckles were missing, and wheels burnt crisp with castings cracked or bent. They had hit the street with unimaginable force, and the frame had been slammed by debris. The stretcher had come from inside the World Trade Center, pulled from the rubble after the towers collapsed. "One of the guys told me they dug it out and used it." He added proudly, "They grabbed whatever they could find. And it still worked. That's how good our product is."

On September 11, 2001, twisted I-beams melted the soles of boots worn by early rescue workers. Police officers dug in the dirt and ashes with their bare hands, with handcuffs, with shards of metal, with a shoe. Twenty people were found alive in what came to be called The Pile. At the periphery, just afterward, civilian volunteers in business suits and women in skirts and heels tended to the injured, clutching water bottles and pressing sodden rags to wounds and burning eyes. Blood trickled into storm sewers.

A total of 2,606 people died that day in New York. In the midst of all this death there were survivors. More than 6,000 were treated for injuries, ranging from cuts and abrasions to broken bones and burns. Rescue tools were scattered amid the gnarled steel and broken glass, silhouetted against the smoke. Cots and trolleys, splints and backboards, litters and basket stretchers moved people away from danger and toward help.

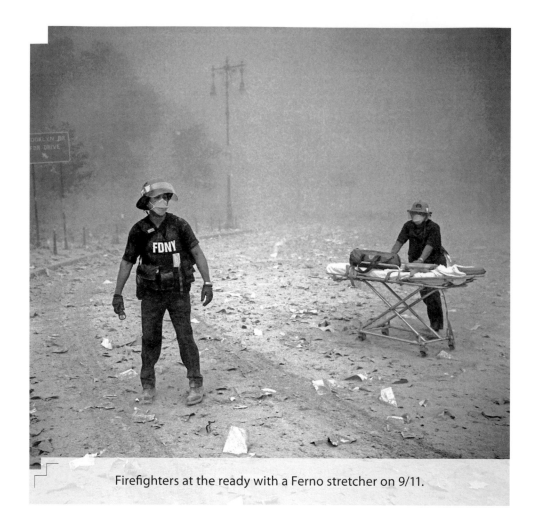

Firefighters at the ready with a Ferno stretcher on 9/11.

Most of this equipment came from Ferno-Washington Inc., the company that invented modern human transport. It is not much of a stretch to conclude that the toll on that September day in America might have been even higher had it not been for the young man's father, Elroy Bourgraf, and his partner, Richard Ferneau. And that the landscape of EMS and rescue services around the world would be very different had the two men not shaken hands in 1956.

Ferno also supplied the means to remove those who died in the towers, a grim duty that is part of this company's DNA. After the attack, searchers climbed the treacherous mountain of ash and steel, writing their names and Social Security numbers on their arms and legs in case they, themselves, needed to be identified later. Another Bourgraf son, Brian, drove to New York in a truck filled with supplies to help them.

"Remains were carried out on what we call our 71 boat, an orange basket," Elroy Jr. said. Workers raked through the wreckage every day for months. "I was there some of the time. When they found something, anything, even a piece of bone, everybody would stop working, cease all activity, take off their hats. They would drape the basket with an American flag and have a brief service. It's an honor to know that all these people were taken out in our baskets."

A chaplain who served there said, "Their reverence was very moving. We're a very physical people. Our bodies are the way we know each other—arms that held us, the shoulder we put our heads on." The two men behind the rescue equipment began their company guided by that same reverence—that respect.

When the heroes of 9/11 raced to save the injured, they used Ferno backboards and stretchers and chairs. They loaded patients into ambulances and rescue vehicles using Ferno cots. It was just as Dick Ferneau envisioned as he sketched obsessively on scratch pads, backs of envelopes, napkins—whatever scrap of paper he could grab when an idea struck. Those who are hurt or sick can travel more safely and comfortably. Those who carry them can work faster, with less wear and tear on their own bodies. His partner, El Bourgraf, translated Dick's designs into equipment that could withstand the rigors of Iceland's winters, Australia's summers, and Germany's regulations.

One partner wrestled with design and function, while the other made these tools available to more than eighty percent of the world. Their passion was to manufacture equipment that is often invisible, folded up and tucked away. Until you need it. And everybody does, sooner or later. Their vision was to think the unthinkable and imagine how it could be better, more tolerable, more dignified—safer.

Pioneering is at once wonderfully different and remarkably the same. Setbacks and triumphs. Treachery and loyalty. Quirky patrons and colorful allies. An absolute confidence in success. Like other American garage entrepreneurs— Steve Jobs, Bill Hewlett and Dave Packard, Walt Disney—El Bourgraf and Dick Ferneau started with more determination than money, substituted nerve and drive for experience, believed they could do something unique, something no one else could or would do, that they could create and lead an industry. And they were right.

The proof is inside nearly every ambulance and hearse on earth.

Handle with Care

Dick Ferneau was a thinker…He would walk down the hall, and he was thinking 100 percent of the time. You might say 'hi' to him, and he would say 'hi' back, but he would never break his pace.

1

The Foundation

El Bourgraf

George Bourgraf sold caskets, and it was not unusual for him to bring his 5-year-old son to the showroom on weekends. The child was so comfortable there, he often snuggled down in one of the plush satin interiors for a nap. "Dad was such a salesman," Elroy said. "When he wasn't attending to a funeral director or a grieving family, he would think of things he could invent to pique their interest, differentiate himself. He even patented a cardboard bra, a fine touch to be used in a casket." George also invented a peel-off funeral flag for cars and a casket for infants. He'd devise projects for his boy, a go-kart or a bird house. Sometimes El and his dad would build them together.

The family moved from the home in Cincinnati where El had been born in 1931 to the suburb of Terrace Park, then back to the city neighborhood of Mt. Airy in 1949, living in a four-family apartment on North Bend Road so El would qualify for city tuition at the University of Cincinnati.

A co-op student, working a series of jobs secured through the university as he earned his degree, he considered this an ideal way to "find out what I didn't want to do in life." He clerked at Shillito's department store and worked in the advertising department at Procter & Gamble for a man by the name of E.A. Snow. "I was exposed to the corporate life, and I saw how tough it was to get to the top. Big company politics was not right for me. I didn't like the culture, the hierarchy, the executive lunchroom."

After making truck bodies for Littleford Brothers on Eastern Avenue, he hustled votes for Bob Taft during "Mr. Republican's" last bid for the Senate. El admired the candidate, the tempo and the decisive people surrounding the campaign, but still wasn't satisfied.

Close but no cigar.

He found the cigar tightly clenched in the teeth of a ladies garment salesman in Cleveland. After notifying UC's placement office that he intended to take charge of his own job arrangements, he drove to Cleveland and invested in a *Plain Dealer*, opening the newspaper to the jobs section.

"I found a job as a bag boy. Well, that's what I called it. I learned to sell ladies ready-to-wear in Ohio, Michigan, Indiana, and Pennsylvania, calling on small-town stores with a short, fat Jewish guy named Herman Englander. Went up on a Saturday, got a job on Sunday and left for Alpena, Pennsylvania, on Monday." They sold ladies' All Season Coats and Suits by Betty Jean of worsted gabardine that the brochure promised would be "A perfect companion for your busy life."

"At first I stayed in the YMCA but later he trusted me in the hotel with him, playing gin rummy and talking business." Herman used to brag to customers about his young assistant. Honest and dependable, he called him. El praised Herman Englander as a professional traveling salesman, who taught him "the tricks of the trade that can make a good salesman a super salesman."

"After we finished the day, we'd drive to the town where we had our next appointment because you never knew what the weather was going to do. We'd find an inexpensive hotel or motel nearby. I'd get up first, real early. While Herman was getting ready, I'd drive his big Cadillac to the store where we had our appointment and park it in front. Then I'd go back, have breakfast and we'd walk to the store. We'd not only be on time but all our stuff would be right outside. So we looked organized."

Then the bag boy would unload the merchandise from the back of the shiny luxury car. Herman had removed the back seats and everything was neatly stacked there. They looked organized. And prosperous.

"I learned his routine, could hand him what he wanted without a word from him. I could see when a buyer liked a certain suit or dress, then I would be ready with coordinates in color and styles." Herman, a gifted salesman, could keep eye contact with the customer as garments magically appeared in his hand. "He'd hold up a ladies dress on a hanger, elbow crooked, his arm extended so you could imagine the way it would drape from her bust line." The bag boy was honest, dependable and had an instinct for selling.

Better. Much better. But still not something El could imagine doing for the rest of his life. Selling was fun, and he knew he had the knack. But he did not see women's ready-to-wear as his destiny. Too much cloth, not enough moving parts. Since the days when he followed his handyman father around, he'd been fascinated with building, with mechanics, with problem solving. Outgoing and curious, he could converse politely with his father's adult clients. Even more helpful, he learned to listen.

As his college career wound down, young El Bourgraf found himself in 1954 with a degree from the University of Cincinnati in business administration, a fierce

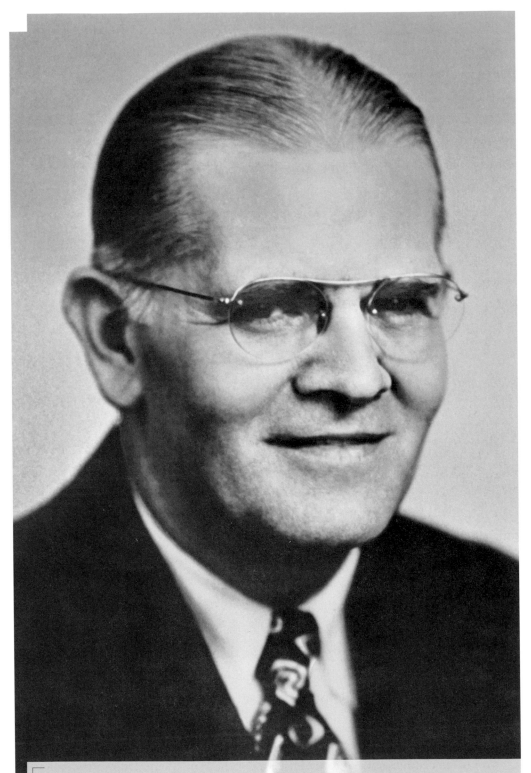

George Bourgraf, a role model and a connection.

work ethic and energy to burn. Not to mention a firm grasp of what he didn't want to do. Thanks to UC's co-op program and his own restless ambition, he had an unusually broad work experience and a whiff of success. He'd sold Fuller Brushes to housewives in the walkable area around the University of Cincinnati, making about $100 a week—pretty good money back then—to supplement what his parents were able to contribute to his tuition and expenses. President and treasurer of his Beta Theta Pi Fraternity, he'd marched with the ROTC cadets on campus and kept his nose in a book long enough to get good but not outstanding grades.

During one of El's college co-op rotations, George Bourgraf had pointed his son toward a business connection, funeral director Burt Weil. El was hired to sell Weil's latest invention, the Slide Under Body Lift, a stretcher rigged with straps which allowed easier handling of a body. The device, which sold for $29.95, cost $10 to make. Burt and El split the profit. It was a good deal.

More than that, Burt launched El on a course that shaped the rest of his life.

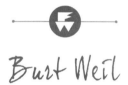

Burt Weil

At the southeast edge of Wilmington, Ohio, in the shadow of the town's squat water tank, is the world headquarters of Ferno-Washington, Inc. The vintage FW logo on a modest square tower is reinforced with a sleek stainless steel Ferno sign at ground level, on the way to the handsome brown brick entry. The address is 70 Weil Way, tangible gratitude from a company whose management is deeply respectful of its human history.

Born in 1897 in Cincinnati, Burt Weil was best known in his hometown as the scion of the mortuary family. But he came to that career by way of a colorful array of interests and accomplishments. His patents included one for bottling citrus of magnesia and another for the first chocolate milk drink. "The funeral business," he told a *Cincinnati Enquirer* reporter in 1973, "started just about the same time Dad turned down the opportunity to purchase the first Coca-Cola franchise." Isaac Weil, who owned a livery service, instead founded Weil Funeral Home in 1912.

Young Burt bought and sold rental horses and the team that pulled the company hearse, working with his older brothers, Sidney and Gordon. When the automobile came along, the brothers bought a New York mineral water operation and started the Grand Pop Bottling Company to take advantage of Burt's chocolate and citrus drinks. Sold and resold, Grand Pop was an early Pepsi franchise. Collectors today will pay $50 for a bottle from that era sporting the Pepsi logo and the Grand Pop stamp. The enterprising Weils branched out into furniture and baseball, with controlling interest at one time in the Cincinnati Reds. Then they were smacked by the Depression.

Sid, the eldest, turned his considerable acumen to the automotive and insurance industries. Gordon and Burt were back in the funeral business. A man of immense dignity and charm, Burt thought a good deal about the "funeral experience," one most of us take for granted. Wide, soft rubber wheels in swivel casters that would roll quietly and easily on carpeting added to the solemnity of the event just as surely as carefully selected music and an eloquent eulogy. No squeaking, no fumbling. And, to Burt, the experience for the family—and for the company—began when the call came to pick up the deceased.

Fond of saying, "You can always find a helping hand at the end of your arm," Burt sat down and started to think and doodle, his only engineering training from commercial courses at Hughes High School. Later, at the University of Cincinnati, he met his first wife, Olga Strashun, an outstanding college tennis player and golfer. After graduation they lived in North Avondale, an area of Cincinnati then as now, distinguished by its grand architecture, large trees and spacious lots.

Olga continued to compete in both sports, winning several state and local titles. Of course, she needed a huge car to tote around her golf clubs and tennis racquets. When she didn't need it, she tossed the keys to her Plymouth station wagon to the young student peddling her husband's Slide Under Body Lift to area morticians. He made good use of the car, traveling in ever widening circles to demonstrate the device.

He would just hop in the car and go. No appointments. Funeral directors had a lot of down time between services, he reasoned. "I'd just knock on the door, and if they were busy, I'd come back. It was a slam dunk sale, once they saw how it worked," El said. "When other sales people saw it, they wanted to sell it too. So we'd sign them up as distributors."

Burt had formed a mail-order house with his nephew, Harold Weil, and their Chappell Equipment Company handled the billing, shipping and accounting.

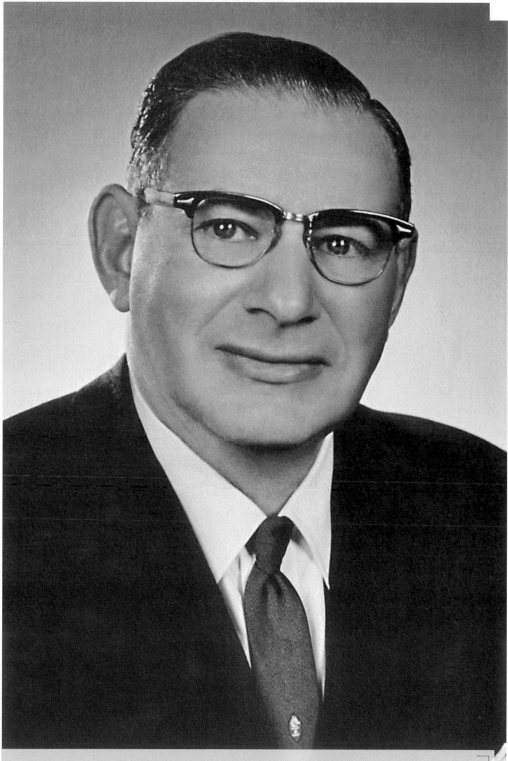

Burt Weil, a good deal that got even better.

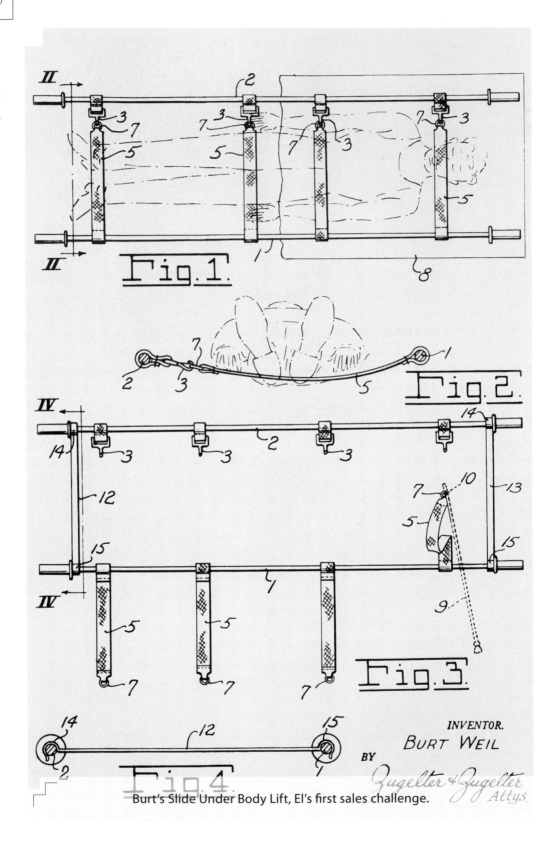

Fig.1.

Fig.2.

Fig.3.

Fig.4.

INVENTOR.
BURT WEIL

BY

Zugelter & Zugelter
Attys.

Burt's Slide Under Body Lift, El's first sales challenge.

Until El came along, the firm had been stumbling along with two or three orders a week. Suddenly business was booming. But the Army had other plans for Chappell's star salesman.

In 1954, the newly graduated El Bourgraf was notified that his presence was required at Fort Bliss, near El Paso, Texas. He dodged live ammo during training and endured dust storms and cramped quarters without complaint, hoping that his next billet might be in Hawaii. After three months, Bourgraf drove his maroon two-door Ford sedan east and, days later, climbed on a troop ship headed for Germany, where he'd spend the next two years.

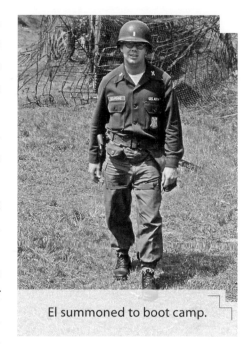

El summoned to boot camp.

He left behind a girl, a job, and the man who would be his most important business partner.

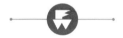

Dick Ferneau

William E. Klever, founder of Washington Mortuary Supply Company, did two very smart things: he invented the first all-aluminum ambulance cot in 1926 and he hired Richard H. Ferneau.

Born in 1919, Dick lived most of his life in Ohio's Fayette Co., the county abutting Clinton to the east. After graduating from high school in 1937, he took a job pumping gas for $11.25 a week. Two weeks later, Bill Klever asked him to try out for a job at his Washington Mortuary Supply Company in Washington Court House, where they sold caskets and made grave markers. Hedging his bets, Dick worked both jobs.

After getting paid $17 for two weeks of evenings and weekends, he signed on full time with Bill, who bumped up his weekly salary to match the one he was

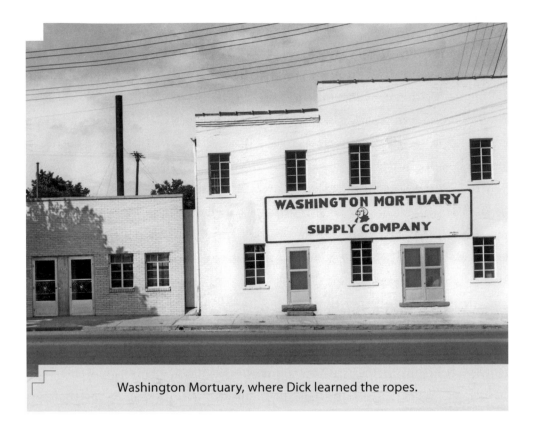

Washington Mortuary, where Dick learned the ropes.

making at the gas station. "I thought there might be a future there," Dick would say. Although he didn't ask, Bill soon gave the young man a 25-cent raise. He worked with the boss, but "the office was not that busy, so I had to work in the plant quite a bit and in the shipping room." Without being asked, he simply did whatever looked like it needed doing.

"My parents, while they were the best," Dick wrote to a friend, "didn't insist on my going on for further education or to church. I remained a clod. I only knew I had to work and make my way."

During World War II, Dick served from 1942 to 1945 in the Army in Corozal, three miles north of Panama City, Panama. He was a patriot, to be sure, but it was also true that Washington Mortuary was unable to get allotments for aluminum and materials and was forced to close during the war years. Bill Klever took a job as a security guard, while the Bomgardner Company in Cleveland won the contract to supply cots for the Army.

At the height of the war, 65,000 American soldiers were stationed in Panama, plus tens of thousands of civilian employees and other military personnel. In spite of the heavy defenses, and the canal's importance to the Allied war effort, Panama never came under attack by the Axis. Dick returned home unscathed and when asked about his Panama adventure, he said, "Hot."

He took up where he left off at Washington Supply, which had moved to a larger building and shifted most of the business toward manufacturing Bill's aluminum cot. Klever died in 1947. By then Dick had a thorough grounding in the mortuary business. And he had ideas.

The widow Klever asked Dick what he thought she ought to do with the company. He said he hoped she'd keep the plant open, that he could see plenty of opportunities for new products. M.Z.—nobody knew what the initials stood for—gave Dick the title of general manager and a fairly loose rein to run the shop. In 1949, he reported a total income of $4,495.30 to the IRS. Mrs. Klever paid the bills and counted the money. He did everything else. And, like Burt Weil, he doodled.

Working with Reynolds Aluminum, Dick came up with smaller, telescoping tubing that he used on the Model 21 Cot, which was not only lighter than anything else on the market but better looking and stronger. Besides reducing the weight of the cot by more than 30 percent, the smaller frame was easier to grasp and carry. Dick took it to trade shows, where he listened to funeral directors complaining about moving patients from their beds at home onto the ambulance cots. In 1952, Washington Mortuary Company introduced its first elevating cot at the National Funeral Directors convention, giving them exactly what Dick had heard them ask for—a smooth, safe, easy transfer from home bed to cot without significant lifting.

"It attracted a lot of attention and made non-elevating cots obsolete," he wrote in a company memo many years later.

Dick might have used the disparaging term, "clod," on himself, but the funeral directors and businessmen in his expanding orbit believed he was something else entirely—honest, resourceful, inventive. Some of them called him a genius.

His Model 52, which would lead to the H-frame cot, took another little bite out of the Bomgardner Company, which had dominated the cot industry since Joseph Bomgardner pioneered wheeled stretchers in 1910. The new Washington Mortuary model could be adjusted to bed levels from thirteen inches to twenty-four, the level of a bed in someone's home and quickly became the standard of the industry. As Emergency Medical Services (EMS) developed in the 1950s and trauma patients were transported directly to the hospital, Emergency Medical Technicians (EMT) needed a cot that would reach to the height of a hospital emergency room stretcher. Dick and engineer Burt Selig answered with the Model 54, which went up to thirty inches—a little higher, a little sturdier and another bite out of the Bomgardners' business in Cleveland.

Meanwhile, funeral directors were beginning to relinquish the transport of the living to fire departments and municipal and private ambulance services. Demand for the combination hearse/ambulance custom coach declined, replaced by station wagons and suburban-type trucks and ultimately the "box" or modular ambulance. The station wagon ambulance was the cheapest, fastest way to get into the transport business, but offered little maneuvering room to attend to a living patient. Dick reacted with the Washington #21L and #54L cots, designed to gain additional space for the attendants.

"I was running the plant and doing purchasing and all of the advertising and the designing and making the shows," he wrote. Perhaps because the Klevers had hired Dick when he wasn't much more than a boy, M.Z. treated him as a combination plant foreman, handyman and chauffeur. He chaffed at her demands and felt under appreciated.

"On June 21, 1955, I had a personal argument with Mrs. Klever and by 10 in the morning I was on my way home without a job. I had no intention of leaving and had no thought in my mind to go prior to that time. I just figured it was eighteen years. Out the window."

He may have left his job without a golden parachute, but he departed with something of great value. Experience and a reputation.

Not even two weeks went by before Dick got a phone call from a man he'd met through conventions and professional association meetings over that eighteen years. Leo Hodroff started working in the family mortuary business at age 13 and graduated from the University of Minnesota in 1939 with a degree in mortuary science. While still in college, he borrowed $100 to launch a mail-order company from the basement of his family's funeral home, selling embalming chemicals and equipment to funeral homes, churches, and schools across the country.

Always impeccably dressed and well spoken, Hodroff was just a couple of years older than Dick and had an impressive reputation of his own. The first

Jewish funeral home director licensed in Minnesota, Leo and his father owned and operated funeral homes at several locations in Minneapolis and St. Paul, the only exclusively Jewish funeral homes in the state. "He was a man of his word," said the rabbi who officiated at Hodroff's funeral service in 2009. She described him as "an honest man with incredible integrity. He had very high standards for himself and for everyone else."

Perhaps Hodroff recognized a kindred entrepreneurial spirit and certainly would have known of Dick's honorable and hardworking nature from his mortuary

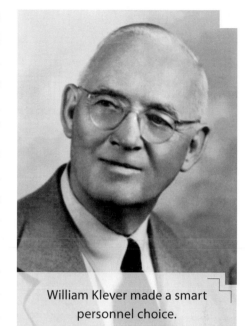

William Klever made a smart personnel choice.

brethren. He was also aware of Dick Ferneau's innovations in the historically static mortuary industry. He pleaded with Dick Ferneau to stay in the business. "I don't want to get into manufacturing," he told Dick, "but I think that's where you belong." He shepherded Dick through the incorporation process, loaned him start-up money and promised to put his products in his Kelco Catalog, which went to virtually every funeral director in the country.

He advised Dick to name his company Ferno Manufacturing Company. "Nobody knows how to spell your name," he said. "And, if they do, they aren't sure how to pronounce it."

The newly minted corporation president came back to Ohio and rented a garage, in the little town of Staunton, Ohio, about seven miles southwest of M.Z's plant in Washington Court House. He developed and started a service to convert existing old low cots into elevating cots. As promised, Leo Hodroff handled the advertising and made sure the service was featured prominently in his catalog. Funeral homes shipped cots to Ohio, where Ferno added elevating mechanisms and sent them back.

"I had only one employee," Dick said. "He could make patterns and operate any type of machine, just the type of man that I needed. We bought some used machinery, a couple of lathes and a drill press, and we were ready to grow."

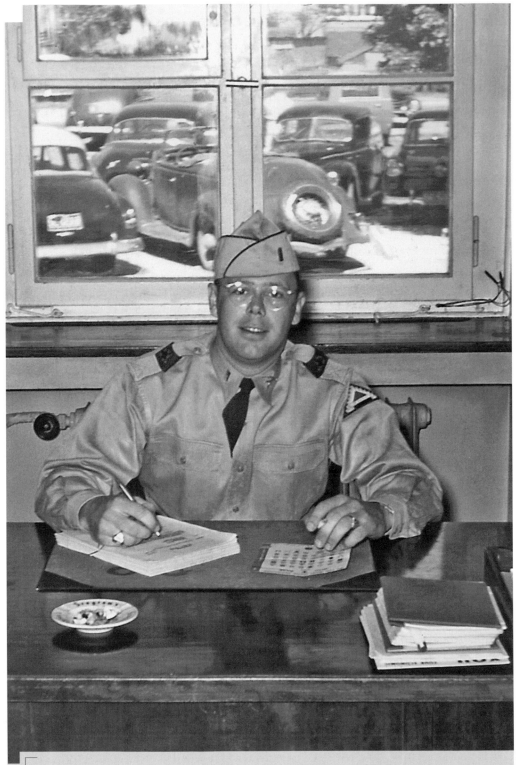

In Germany, the future CEO discovers a taste for leadership.

Just in time for Burt Weil's latest invention.

The funeral director and inventor was looking for a way to make it possible for a single attendant to collect a body for transport to the mortuary. In the fall of 1955, he invented a contraption with bicycle wheels that could be rolled in and out of a funeral car. Sort of. Weil's One-Man Cot was unsightly and ungainly, but when he showed it to Dick, the entrepreneur/engineer immediately grasped the potential. He retooled his elevating cot with longer legs, smaller wheels and a folding undercarriage.

In April 1956, Ferno Manufacturing vacated the Staunton garage and set up shop in a bigger place a few miles east in Circleville. "The One-Man Cot had really taken hold. We were manufacturing just one model, the Model 20. It was strictly for mortuary use and just exactly what the undertakers needed. So many times they had to go out on a call and round up somebody just to help them lift the cot in and out of the car," Dick recalled.

Then Burt Weil, who had presented Dick Ferneau with the prototype of his company's first important product, sent him somebody who could sell it.

El and Dick

By the time El Bourgraf came home from Germany, after finishing non-wartime duty in the Army, he was ready for his real life to start.

First of all, there was The Girl. The lovely Elaine Kunkel of the storied pickle and sauerkraut family, mainstays of Cincinnati's historic Findlay Market for more than 150 years, was not exactly waiting. But she had not forgotten him. Sitting on a couch in the Beta Theta Pi house in 1953 at the University of Cincinnati, she'd noticed the tall, handsome president of the fraternity. El Bourgraf was organizing a weekend event with Elaine's Theta Phi Alpha sisters. Soft-spoken, yet clearly in charge.

A prominent man, he was nonetheless, rather graceful with a purposeful walk. He would never be the one to stumble through a room and bump into the coffee table. And never, ever would he be the one with a lampshade on his head.

"I hope he calls me. I hope he calls me," she said to herself.

He did. Two or three dates. But he was headed for graduation, then a troop ship.

Two years later, on his first Sunday back home, he went to church with his parents in Mt. Airy. "I caught his eye in the parking lot," Elaine remembers. She also remembers keeping her gloves on because they covered an engagement ring. She broke off her half-hearted engagement to another man and repeated the pre-feminist mantra from her college days: "I hope he calls me. I hope he calls me." And waited.

"That young man with the funny name telephoned again," her mother would tell her. El repeated the courtus-interruptus of his college days. They went out, but El stopped calling because "I couldn't afford anything." He meant to change that.

When El was stationed at the military base in Karlsruhe, Germany, near the French border, building up his Chesterfield cigarette habit to four packs a day and commanding an anti-aircraft battery, he considered staying in the Army. "Maybe it was a little bit of the macho in me, but I know I liked the discipline and the challenge." As when he'd led his fraternity in college, he enjoyed being in charge of the troops. He just wasn't sure the Army would allow him to avoid jobs he didn't like to do. And his unwavering aim was to find a position where he could do less of what he didn't like and more of what he did.

"Money was never the primary motivation for me," he would say, long after he had enough of it. "As Burt Weil used to say, you can only eat one steak at a time, drive one Cadillac."

Letters from home included one from Burt that contained a picture of a mortuary cot. "It was a monstrosity," El remembered, laughing. "This was before Dick Ferneau got ahold of it."

Burt's primitive-looking prototype in Dick Ferneau's hands became the Ferno 20 One-Man Mortuary Cot. El liked selling, and he liked the mortuary business. Understood it. After a gentle nudge or seven from George Bourgraf, he spurned an offer from Procter & Gamble and in July of 1956 agreed to sell Burt Weil's latest invention, taking up where he'd left off at Chappell Equipment. Burt sent him out to the plant to meet the manufacturer.

"While at Circleville, Burt Weil sent El Bourgraf up to me," Dick said. "Burt figured that the two of us would make a pretty good team."

El and Dick thought the same thing, almost right away. El likes to call instant, instinctive human connections "chemistry." Dick would say later that "we could

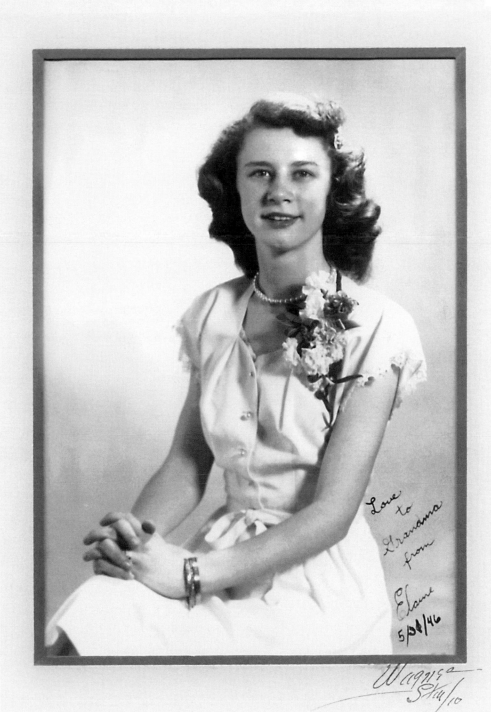

Elaine Kunkel in 1946, the girl El left behind.

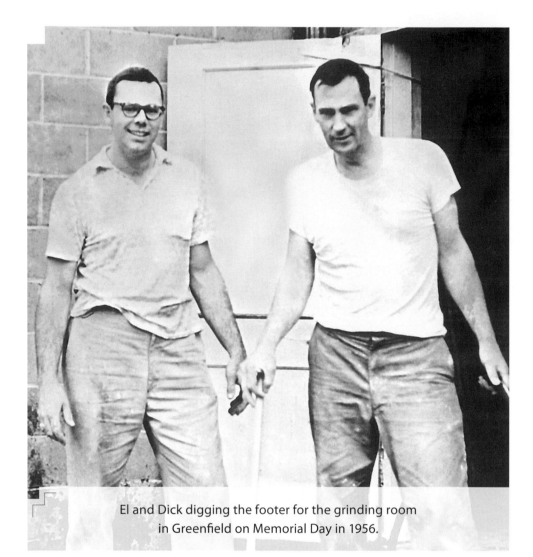

El and Dick digging the footer for the grinding room
in Greenfield on Memorial Day in 1956.

see we needed each other as far as something for the future." They became partners
by the end of 1956. They were alike in the ways that mattered and different in ways
that strengthened them both.

El cleaned up a few outstanding debts Dick owed, money he'd borrowed to get
started. "Not a whole lot of money," El said. "And at that point Ferno wasn't making
enough to keep the lights on."

He moved to Circleville, and the two men routinely worked twelve-hour days,
starting at 6:30 in the morning, "until we got the business pretty well cranked
up." El was starting to put his business degree to good use, and Dick had the
machinery humming.

"Dick Ferneau was a thinker," according to Ellen Coleman, who has worked at Ferno for thirty-seven years, most of them as a machinist. "He would walk down the hall, and he was thinking 100 percent of the time. You might say 'hi' to him, and he would say 'hi' back, but he would never break his pace. He'd stop in mid-stride because he thought of something else, and he'd turn around. And he might do that three or four times in three minutes because, he was just always thinking. He was a very, very humble man. He didn't want anything to do with any of the business part. He just wanted to design, to build. That was his passion. His attitude was 'Just let me loose to build things.'"

It was the classic business partnership—the inside man and the outside man. The more introverted Dick Ferneau still maintained strong ties with the customers who'd given him ideas to ponder and turn into aluminum tubes, straps and wheels, but he was only really comfortable with them one at a time. "He was a loner," El said. And Dick most loved being alone with a scrap of paper and the stub of a pencil.

Dick's title was general manager, and he was the nominal head of R&D. But titles weren't important to either of them.

The more extroverted El, who was in charge of marketing and sales, carried a crisp business card with the company name and his own. No title. And just as Dick had done when he started working with Bill Klever, they both simply did whatever looked like it needed doing. El worked in the grinding room and machine shop and assembled cots. Aluminum castings came in rough, needing a polish. It was dirty business, standing over a buffing wheel in the grinding room. Noisy. "I've never asked people to do anything I wasn't willing to do," El says. And he never says somebody worked for him. They worked *with* him. It was not just words.

Fueled by sales of the One-Man Cot, the company outgrew its Circleville location. They moved to larger quarters thirty miles away in Greenfield, Ohio, on June 21, 1957. Close enough for employees to follow if they wanted. Most of them did.

In the boardroom of Ferno-Washington's headquarters at 70 Weil Way is an eight-by-ten black and white photo of the company's founders, looking decidedly unlike executives, in stained tee-shirts and wrinkled work pants, sweaty, digging the footer for the grinding room in Greenfield on Memorial Day in 1956. They would build the foundation of their company together, as surely and as unpretentiously as they did that footer.

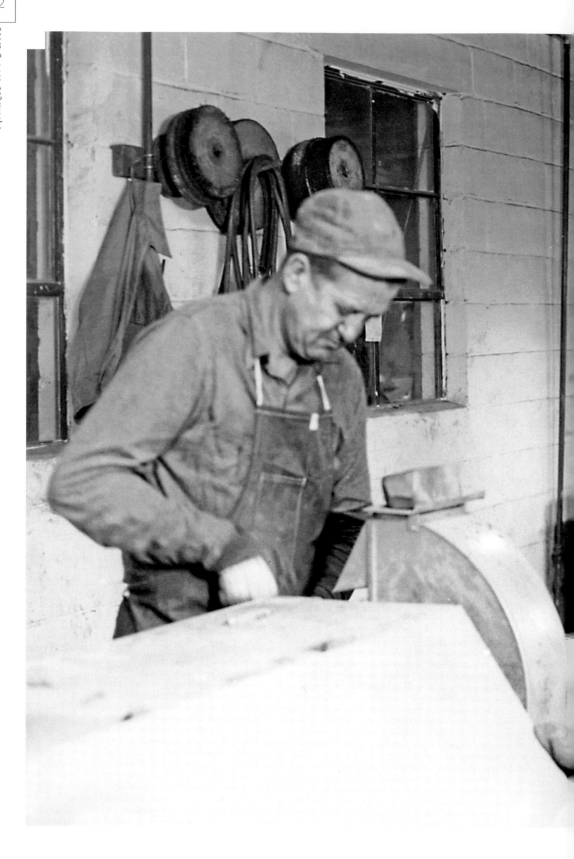

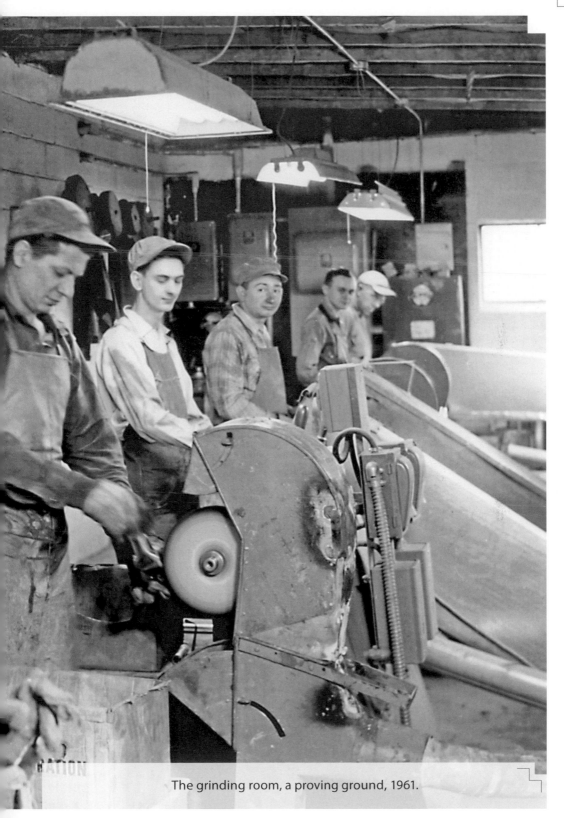

The grinding room, a proving ground, 1961.

It was the genesis of this company's culture—respect and a leeway to create and speak freely. Add to that, an appreciation of the human beings who would be on the cot and the ones who would be carrying it…

2

The Partnership

INVALEX CO INC.

Gearing Up in Greenfield

When Elaine Kunkel Bourgraf gave birth to her first son, some of the neighbors heard the good news before her husband did. Oh, El was around, pacing a little, but mostly sitting on a butt-sprung couch outside swinging hospital doors that separated him from his wife's labors. There were outdated magazines and ashtrays for nervous dads-to-be. But no telephone.

This was the day of the party line and Ma Bell's operators who trilled *Numbrrrr pleeeze* when you picked up the phone. Every phone call came through a switchboard operator, and several households shared a line. Eavesdropping was a way of life, the original reality show. Phone operators knew just about everything that was happening in the little town of Greenfield and with party lines, so did everybody else. "It was common for people to dial the operator to locate someone," El said. "I think the operator was the one who tracked me down to let me know it was time for Elaine to go to the hospital. And, somehow, I think the phone company got the word first of Joe's birth. Small towns. I love 'em. Always have."

Ferno moved in June of 1957 to Greenfield, a community situated mostly in Highland County with a toe in neighboring Fayette and Ross counties. A Ferno newsletter to employees promised: "Greenfield is a typical small southern Ohio town. Lots of trees. Lots of kids and dogs—all friendly. The grownups are good natured, neighborly, and don't give a hang about the jet set, Zen Buddhism, or keeping up with the Joneses. Greenfield people believe in doing a job right the first time."

Populated by about 4,500 people, the town's motto is "A Perfect Place to Raise a Family." For those first few years, "family" for Dick and El meant the employees at Sixth and Pine streets, who were fabricating an expanded line of ambulance cots, emergency stretchers, and mortuary tables, as well as safety belts, cot fasteners, foam mattresses, body bags and covers.

At first, it "was hand-to-mouth," El remembered, adding that his take home pay was $75 a week, "assuming all the checks came in the mail." The men worked long hours, and business grew steadily. "Neither Dick nor I ever thought we would fail." The year Dick and El began their partnership, Dun & Bradstreet reported a net worth of $25,000, limited working funds, and a good payment record.

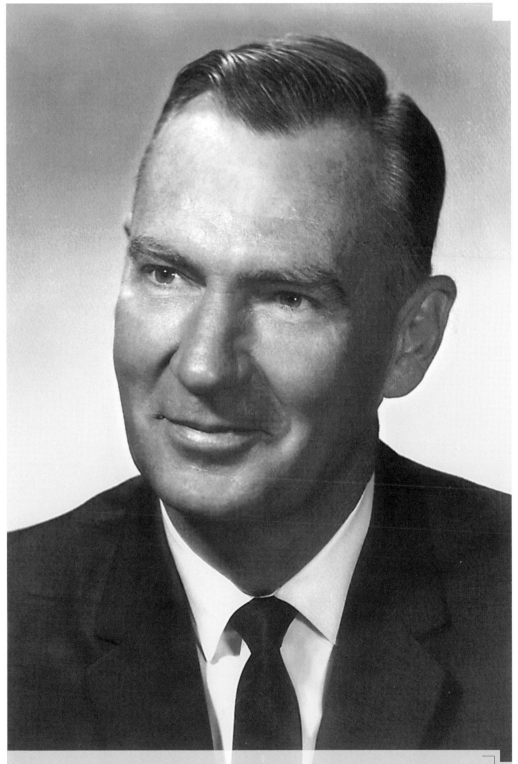

Dick was impatient to put new ideas to work.

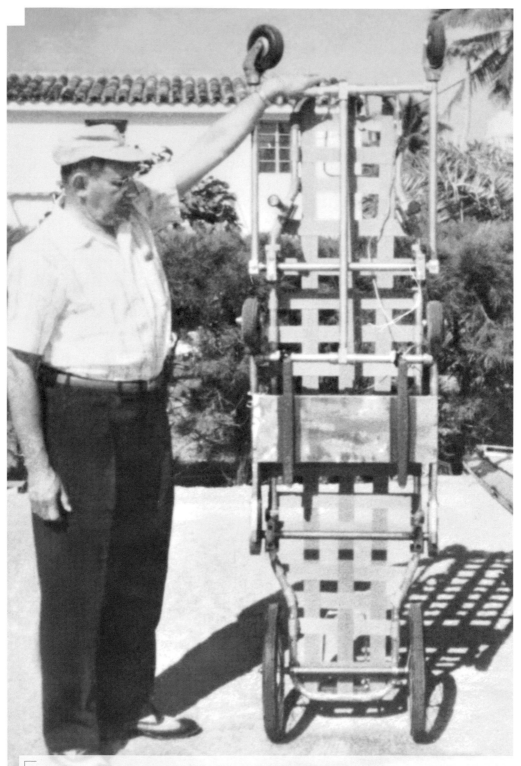

Burt Weil with the One-Man Cot, star of the show.

A year later, D&B noted, "Strong demand for company's principal product has resulted in a 300 percent increase in sales over a nine-month period, approximately $25,000 monthly. Total assets were recorded at $70,000."

As his prospects improved, El found time, finally, to woo and marry Elaine in February of 1960. The ceremony took place on George Washington's birthday, a Monday, chosen because the pickle stand would be closed for the holiday, but never on a Saturday. No doubt reassuring those listening on the party line and counting, Joe was not born until November of that

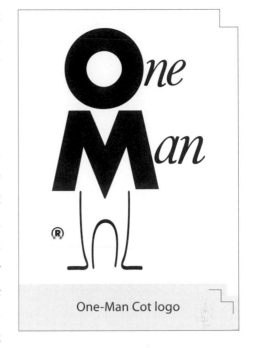

One-Man Cot logo

year. El managed to successfully juggle both his Ferno family and his growing Bourgraf family, but he was spending more time on the road, selling.

"We had a product that lasted a long time and were marketing to buyers who didn't need a whole lot of them. We had to expand our horizons, geographically," El said. They also expanded the product line.

Burt Weil's One-Man Mortuary Cot was still the star of the show, selling for $199.50, including pad and straps. The literature addressed pressing concerns of those in the profession. "Here is a cot that enables one man to make a first call, eliminates most of the dangerous physical strain, allows more evenings free and more uninterrupted sleep, and eases employment problems." Furthermore, the brochures observed, the cot "allows more time for personal service to the family of the deceased and provides new dignity."

The biggest advantage, El would say with his customary honesty was it "saved the guys' backs."

El described the mechanism, which would be the inspiration for many future products: "The attendant rolls the cot to the open coach. When the large forward wheels make contact with the rear of the coach, the attendant releases the undercarriage with his knee and the coach assumes half the weight of the cot and patient while the attendant supported the other half as he pushes it into the vehicle."

Marketing was making a decided pivot, with more references to patients and emphasis on emergency products for the ambulance. Ferno still proudly displayed its mortuary cot and stainless steel embalming table and introduced a space-saving folding embalming table, while continuing to do a brisk business selling body bags and elegant covers, as well as church and showroom trucks to move and display caskets.

The staff back in Greenfield was expanding to fill El's shoes while he was on the road and to give him time with his family. Ferno introduced the Model 25 ambulance version of the One-Man Mortuary Cot, and shortly after the Model 30 All-Level cot and the Model 108 Stretch'r Chair, a portable cot with a chair back were added to the product line.

"It got a lot of attention and brought in a lot of orders." Dick wrote in correspondence preserved in Ferno's archives. "We were rapidly getting ahead of other dealers but felt like we were hurting the Washington Mortuary business. In 1960, El and I thought we should try to purchase Washington Mortuary Supply from Mrs. Klever. We knew she was struggling."

They finalized the deal in 1961, and the company officially became Ferno-Washington, Inc. in 1963. Mrs. Klever maintained her home in Washington Court House until her death at 91. The name carved on her tombstone is M.Z. Klever, and the old two-story brick Washington Mortuary building a few streets over was torn down to make way for the Country Mark Feed Plant.

El later negotiated another acquisition, a cemetery tent manufacturer in Pikesville, Ky. Teletent didn't make much money, but Ferno management was getting a taste of growth through acquisition. Then, in rapid succession, Ferno introduced the Model 27, allowing patients to sit up inside low headroom cars, and the Model 32, an elevating Stretch'r Cot with a recessing bed.

By 1962, product lines included one-man cots, two-level cots, cot fasteners, Model 11 folding lightweight stretcher, Model 40 folding stair chair, Model 46 aircraft invalid loading chair, Model 107 combination stretcher-chair, and Model 104 telescoping stretcher series.

Next came the Model 28 Fernoflex ambulance chair-cot, a huge success and a game changer. It is still the only full ambulance cot that converts to a chair. The advance in design and technology was nearly equal in importance to the One-Man Cot or the X-frame all-level cot, according to El, who introduced the product in

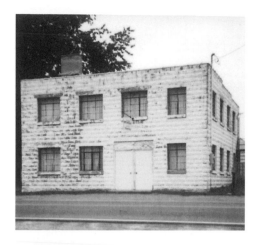

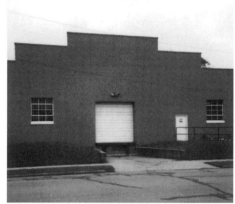

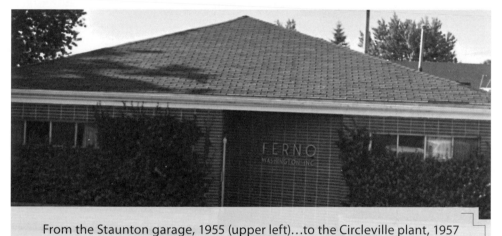

From the Staunton garage, 1955 (upper left)…to the Circleville plant, 1957 (upper right)…to the Greenfield headquarters.

November of 1964. EMTs had been telling him that chronic back pain was their most serious work-related problem, and they immediately recognized the new product as a solution to chronic challenges such as carrying patients down narrow staircases, and coping with tight spaces in elevators and hallways, thus making it one of the most widely used products in the world today.

The Scoop Stretcher, an idea from El that was both simple and elegant, would also survive for a half century—with minor tweaks—and can be found in virtually every ambulance in the world today. Like giant cupped metal and plastic hands that slide gently under dazed quarterbacks or accident victims, they help move people without contributing to their injuries. At roadside accident scenes, "Attendants can readily uncouple either or both ends to gently scoop the injured onto the stretcher, eliminating rolling, sliding, twisting or lifting the victim," read the catalog introducing the scoop in 1965. El likes to describe it simply as "working like a pair of scissors."

By 1967, the One-Man Mortuary Cot for funeral homes represented less than 17 percent of sales.

El attended EMS conventions while carefully maintaining long-standing relationships with funeral directors. Models 86 and 87, the first new church models in fifty years, added length and stability, while still conveniently folding up to fit inside a hearse. The new equipment also added subtle dignity to an otherwise grim ordeal, providing new choices in appearance and finish. It looked contemporary, and underscored Ferno's commitment to its mortuary market. "Business 101," El said. "Don't neglect the customers you have while you are getting new ones."

On a road trip, El observed a procedure in an embalming room. The woman on the stainless steel Ferno table had been a heavy smoker. Her lungs were black. El, still a four-pack-a-day man, threw away his cigarettes. Temporarily. Cranky but determined, he made Elaine and his secretary, Millie Head, gatekeepers of the nicotine. "They made it difficult for me to light up," he said. Then impossible.

El's doctor told him his lungs probably looked like the cadaver he'd seen. Black. "But he told me they could be pink again in a couple of years. Thinking of that helped me when Elaine and Millie weren't around, when I was traveling," El said. Plus, he and Elaine now had another son, Brian, suffering from a rare and debilitating array of birth defects. El's responsibilities were getting more complicated both at home and at work.

Dick and El agreed to take the long view, selling to wholesale outlets only, cementing relationships with distributors.

A memo went out: "The decision is positive evidence of our confidence in the ability of you and your salesmen to develop and secure the sales volume. We will support your efforts with an enlarged national advertising program."

Working *with* them. Other partnerships, of sorts.

El's language toward his co-workers and his customers was "not just lip service," as Dick would say. The company's genuine respect for its growing roster of partners drew the Ferno family together over many decades and through tense growing pains, including a determined pitch by labor union organizers.

Lifting as They Climb

Ellen Coleman, the machinist who started at Ferno when she was just out of high school, slipped on the ice a few years ago at her home. Still conscious and ever sensible, she called 911. "When the EMTs got there, I was bent over, and out of the corner of my eye I saw our competitor's cot," she said. She refused to get aboard.

"I can't ride on that," she told the EMT. "I work at Ferno." He thought a minute and said, "Well, the backboard's from Ferno."

Mollified, she reconsidered. "Good enough." Coleman said.

Reminiscing about nearly four decades at Ferno, she said, "When I first started, everything was smaller. It was neat. When we had group meetings, El would meet with each department personally." Engineering had lunch with R&D and accounting had potluck dinner with management who took a smoke break with manufacturing. The head of marketing knew how to grind casters. Inspiration for a cot design came when El and Dick were having an after-work beer with a co-worker and her husband. Jane Fox, a secretary/bookkeeper/receptionist and working mom, was comfortable enough with her bosses to drag out an ironing board so she could chat while catching up on the laundry.

They watched her push a release lever as she raised the board all the way up, then adjusted it down to the height she needed to iron her daughter's dress. "We looked at each other," El said, "and Dick and I both had the same idea." A week later, they'd developed the Model 30, the first X-frame all-level cot. It looked a lot like Jane Fox's ironing board.

Fully integrated? You bet. Chemistry? The company was crawling with it. "And that's evolved into this huge company and companies all over the world," Ellen Coleman said. "I have grown up as Ferno has grown up. We've grown up together."

Like Ellen, Irvin Pollock worked at Ferno his entire adult life—beginning as a co-op student his senior year in high school and staying forty-seven more years. "Dick and El worked so close with us they could see our potential. Then we'd move on up in the company. In a large company, you might see the president once in a

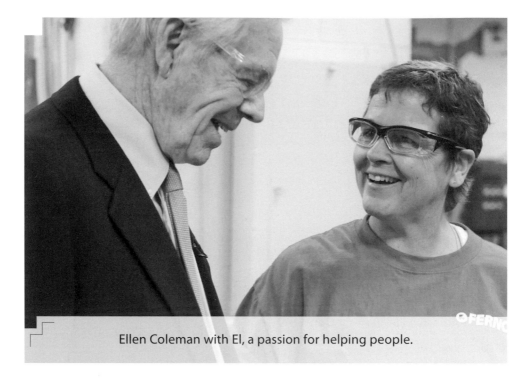

Ellen Coleman with El, a passion for helping people.

blue moon, but they were around and they saw what we were doing, commented on what we were doing. It really, really gives you the boost to get in there and dig and put in 100 percent."

He started at Ferno doing sub-assembly, then worked his way into the machine shop and eventually became one of the key people on the R&D team. "Then I went into specialty work," he said, "where if somebody wanted something a little bit special and different than the standard cut, we would make it."

Sometimes the market for these specialty items was exactly one.

Parents of a little girl came to Ferno asking if somebody could design a walker for their daughter. "Her upper body was normal, but her legs just never grew," remembers Dave Haines, who started working in Greenfield in 1960 and eventually became vice president of manufacturing. The guys in the shop made a small bicycle with four wheels, surrounding it with a railing. "She went to school on it. She went to prom on it. Sent us pictures of her at the prom on her little special walker."

The cost? "Well, we didn't keep a record," El said. "And the bill got lost."

Another time, this "fairly small company" outfitted a van for the wife of an Army veteran paralyzed by a stroke. "He was a big guy, and she wanted to be able to move him around and travel with him," Dave said. "So we built a special cot that would fit in their van and elevated it so he could see forward." Then they mounted a winch so his wife could push her husband's wheelchair to the vehicle, hitch him to the small jib crane, pick him up, put him on the cot. "She could do it herself, and she wasn't a very big woman," Haines said with satisfaction. "Ferno did amazing things like that just because somebody asked. It's an attitude."

A photo of a group of children on a playground crisscrossed by metal rails was posted on the Ferno bulletin board with a note: "Last spring, some of the men in your shop made this set of bars and a table for us to take to a school for crippled children in Columbus. They use this equipment every day. Our thanks for what you have done for these kids who can't walk and can't be outside without these bars to hang on to."

Right after 9/11, Ellen Coleman was asked to speak to a group of sixth graders about first responders. "I took in a big poster of a New York fireman with a Ferno cot. I said, 'I help build these cots.' I'm not building a chair or a pencil. I have a passion for helping people. And when I see things like that, I know I'm helping people."

El's memories of those Greenfield years include a priceless exchange of ideas, a give-and-take he was determined to preserve, even as the company grew.

"Irv Pollock wasn't afraid to question anything," El said. "We welcome that from any employee, because that's how we learn. Irv was a good listener, but when he had something to say, he'd speak up. I always appreciated his ingenuity. You'd give him an idea and tell him how you think it ought to be. Sometimes he found a better way, and he did it. Didn't ask, just did it. That's innovation, initiative, the thing you really try to encourage in everybody, the thing you never want to lose no matter how big you get."

It was the genesis of this company's culture—respect and a leeway to create and speak freely. Add to that, an appreciation of the human beings who would be on the cot and the ones who would be carrying it—the people connected to their work.

"It didn't just happen overnight. It wasn't a preplanned vision. It was an evolution," El said. A half century later, Ferno's new young CEO would call it, "a passion for people and a respect for the care of human beings."

A typical day at the Greenfield plant might begin in what was loosely the Research and Development area. "I'd start there in the morning," El said, "and we'd talk about something, a problem or whatever was going on or maybe just,

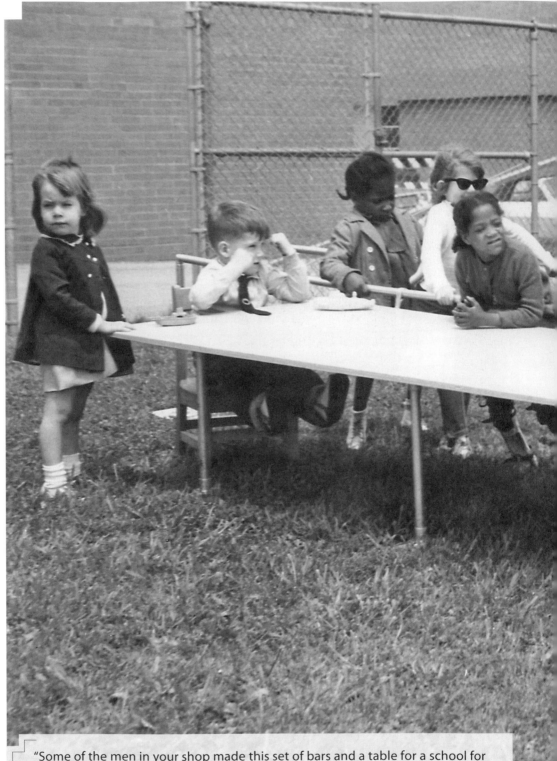

"Some of the men in your shop made this set of bars and a table for a school for crippled children in Columbus. They use this equipment every day," read the note.

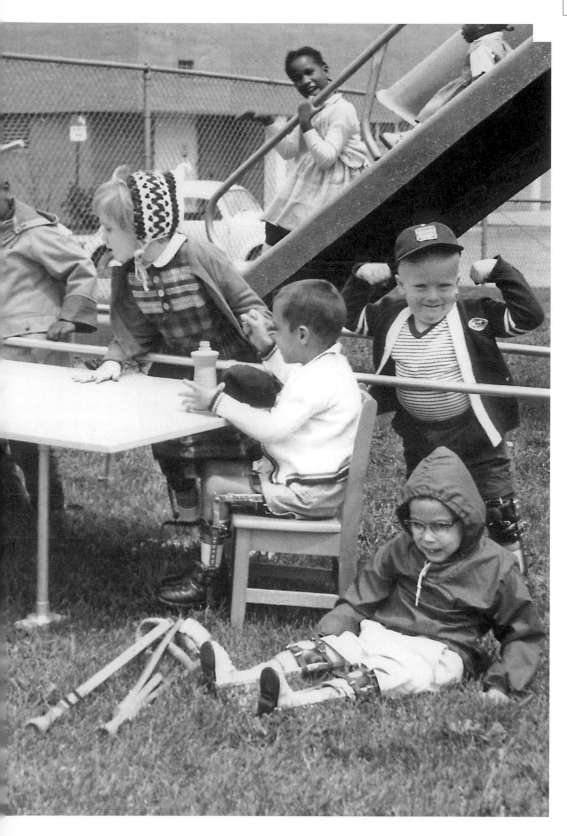

who won the ballgame last night. Last thing in the afternoon, before they'd head home, I'd find a minute or two to get back and ask, 'Okay, what did we do today?'" They knew he was coming and besides the days' work report, they sometimes had figured out the answer to a question from the morning's casual meeting. "El would talk to me about something, ask my opinion," Irvin remembered. "Sometimes, right then, I didn't have an answer for him. But maybe that afternoon or the next day I had thought it through and come up with something."

Once the "something" was the solution for transporting obese patients. El wondered what Irvin thought might be the best bed for the project, suggesting a type of fabric. Irvin had a better idea. "I'm going to put an aluminum bed in it," Irvin said. "And we'll put a nice pad on it," and he said, "Something kind of solid. My wife worked on the life squad and they went to pick up this fellow and he was in a waterbed, and he was totally out." The team of four struggled to wrest him from the undulating surface. "If he had been on something solid, they could have slid him over."

El said, "That's good enough for me."

The 124 casket table is a tubular frame with large rubber rollers that facilitated loading caskets into and out of coaches. Irvin said, "The size of the vehicles kept changing, and so we were making all these special tables of different lengths. I got the bright idea for one we could adjust. That's when I came up with the 124 table."

The boss was impressed. "I liked it. It simplified manufacturing. It was a popular item and a necessary item."

When union organizers approached Ferno employees in the early 1960s, El saw it as a serious menace to the future of the company and to his ability to have these conversations. He went into full business mode. El Bourgraf's habitual decency, soft voice and casual manner are his personal style. He has always run his business with warmth, but definitely not by the seat of his pants and most definitely with a competitor's fierce desire to win.

On Oct. 8, 1963, a memo went out to Ferno-Washington employees over Dick's and El's signatures:

"The Machinists Union has asked for an election at our Greenfield and Washington Court House plants. Because we have faith in our employees' good judgment, we will accept this challenge. We will ask the U.S. Government to supervise this election in which each of you can vote on this union question. Your vote will be the answer to this threat to our friendly relations and job security. More later."

El sought advice from labor relations lawyers and other business owners, and this first salvo was followed a week later by an elaborate outline of the rules of engagement from El and Dick:

"There are certain things the law forbids an employer and supervisory employees to say and do during the period before an election. At the same time, the company and its supervisors have the right of free speech, and there is much the law permits.

"We will tell our employees why we believe this union would not be good for them or for their families and that belonging to this greedy union will cost them lots of money. We will tell our employees that this union cannot guarantee them jobs or job security—that only satisfied customers can provide real job security. We will tell our employees that this outside union is not democratic, that big city bosses run the whole show and care nothing about employees at small plants like ours.

"We won't make any promises of benefits or make any threats to employees if they do or do not vote against the union. We won't tell our employees that our plants will close if the union comes in or that employees will be discharged for supporting the union."

They also promised not to question employees about union activities and ended with:

"The basic rules that will govern what we say boil down to this. We will express our opinion and give true facts. We won't make threats or promises to employees to encourage or discourage union activity."

El started a personal diary as events unfolded, including a report from an employee who was approached at his home by a union representative who offered him a bottle of whiskey and a union card. Ferno's chief kept an eye on activity at the bowling alley and the local motel to see if union recruiters had summoned reinforcements.

Dick Ferneau, who avoided large groups and loathed making speeches, stood up before a gathering of employees in November:

"We've worked hard here trying to build. We've all worked together. We've all worked hard. We are not going to stand by and let the union ruin us. We're going to oppose it with everything we've got. The union can promise you a whole lot, but they can't deliver a thing unless we agree to it. If we give them a great big fat NO and they yell STRIKE and you go through that door, that puts you on the sidewalk."

El followed Dick's remarks with:

"I shouldn't be out here doing this kind of a thing. I would much rather be out selling and putting orders on the books. Don't forget, it's the customer who buys our stuff. A little bit of you is in that. You built it. A little bit of me is in that because I sold it. Never forget that customer.

"I don't think anybody in this group was at the old Washington Mortuary Supply Company. You don't know the way it feels to work for a sick company—to know that awful feeling in the pit of your stomach when there's a helluva a lot less orders on the books than there are people walking around the plant."

The union countered this gathering with an invitation to Ferno employees:

"Now is the time to go after HIGHER WAGES and BIGGER BONUSES. You can bring your wife or girlfriend to this meeting. Lunches and refreshments will be served. It's hootenanny time, so if you play a guitar, banjo or violin or any other type instrument be sure and bring it to the meeting tonight."

A flyer from the machinists' union followed with the testimonial:

"When I think I'm not being treated right on the job, I go to my steward—the guy we elected to take up our complaints with the foreman. And the foreman listens and helps set things right because he knows we're all sticking together. I don't have to keep my mouth shut for fear I'll be fired if I do a little complaining. I don't bottle my anger up inside me all day and come home and take it out on Mary."

Ferno employees declined the opportunity to insert a shop steward between themselves and company owners who not only conferred with them daily but often worked next to them. The union was voted down 41 to 28 in January of 1964.

"For years, I never laid anybody off," El said. "I'd try to keep them working no matter what. And I always leveled with them. From day one, I have shared financial information with everybody. There has always been a bulletin board at the plant where they can look at production numbers."

At the beginning of the year, all employees are made aware of sales and profit goals and are updated quarterly.

A few years later, the union made another run at Ferno. No vote took place. Dave Haines said, "When union guys showed up one day, our people ran them off.

No one told them to. They wanted their company left alone. If there were issues within the company, people wise, peer pressure could usually solve the problem. El wasn't around all the time but I could always call him or contact him." And Dave was confident his boss would listen.

Sometimes, Dave didn't pick up the phone. "I did my job as if the company was mine. There was very little difference between professional and personal here at Ferno. You didn't have to play any games."

A partnership had been forged, as binding as the one between El and Dick, a partnership with many associates, including Dave and Irv and Ellen, and most especially Bernie Zoldak. Unique. Beloved. The guy with a bounce in his walk.

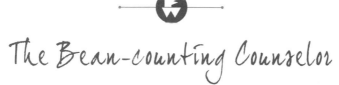

The Bean-counting Counselor

It was chemistry again. "Usually, it doesn't work to hire friends," El mused. "But Bernie was the exception that proved the rule." The two men met in Germany, both new officers, both went to the Catholic Church near the base in Karlsruhe on Sunday, both had grown up in Ohio. Bernie was from Struthers, a town about the size of Wilmington, near Youngstown, where he got his degree in business at the university there. Bernie's wife, Mary Lou, joined him in Germany, and El spent most holidays with the couple at their home.

"When I got tired of living in a sleeping bag, I went home," El said. Bernie stayed behind, planning to make the Army his career. El exchanged Christmas cards with the Zoldaks, who eventually landed back in the states at Fort Sill in Oklahoma. El swung by for a visit after a sales trip out that way. "I sensed that Mary Lou was not totally satisfied, and I thought maybe Bernie might have a future with us."

Bernie finished his four-year Army hitch, and in 1958, the Zoldaks moved to Greenfield, where Bernie accepted a job as Ferno's office manager and purchasing agent. "I had a real need for somebody in administration," El said. "I was on the road all week, then trying to catch up on weekends." Plus, neither he nor Dick really liked counting beans. Dick was a shop man, and El loved meeting clients "getting to know the industry, listening to their problems." El called Bernie "my financial arm and the buffer between me and Dick."

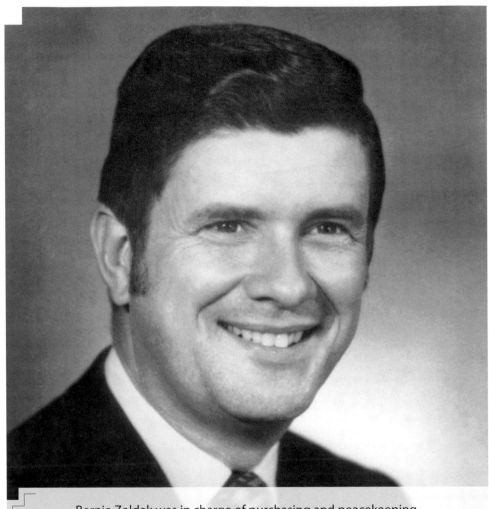

Bernie Zoldak was in charge of purchasing and peacekeeping.

Rather than being wary or jealous of the new guy who had a history with his partner, Dick Ferneau embraced Bernie right away. In a note to Bernie's wife in 1961, Dick wrote, "Poor old Bern has really been putting in the hours—as if you hadn't noticed! I appreciate it more than I can say. It is really over and above the call of duty, but we are all one and working toward the same goal."

Dick trusted Bernie Zoldak, liked him and respected his know-how. Most people did. The new Ferno hire quickly worked himself into community life while he was making himself indispensable around the plant. He joined Greenfield Rotary Club, was a trustee of the Memorial Hospital where two of the Bourgraf sons were born, and served two terms on the City Council.

"So many things just seemed to fall into place with the three of us," El said, beginning to realize his early goal of "doing more of what I like, less of what I didn't."

The man who put his son on this course, who brought his little boy to work with him, then propelled him toward a mentor and a partner, collapsed and died while on a sales call in 1965. George Bourgraf lived long enough to see his son's business flourish and know his role in El's destiny.

In a letter to Dick Ferneau in 1964, George wrote, "I am so thankful that El could have your guidance since he embarked on his career. He has always been dynamic minus the flamboyancy that comes with it, and his association with you has kept him in balance. The results you two have made make my shirt buttons pop, and I would be selfish if I didn't tell you."

Burt Weil was still in the mix, with ideas and advice, collecting royalties and continuing to doodle. Around the shop, they used to call him "Mr. Fabulous." At one point he was in touch with celebrity engineer John DeLorean. "I think Burt was fascinated with the stainless steel car and gull wings," El said.

Sometimes Burt used Bernie to get ideas to Dick and El. More often, Bernie was shuttling back and forth between the partners. Explaining. Soothing. Keeping the peace.

"Dick and I had a unique relationship," El said. "We seldom agreed on anything initially. That was real obvious right from the very start, but we also had a lot of common interests. We both liked to work. We both had a vision of success. We had that in common. We didn't talk to each other much, so that first year, people sometimes thought we were at odds with each other. We weren't. We just had things to do and why waste time talking? We'd leave notes for each other. Maybe out in the shop or on our desks. Or on the windshields of our cars."

About anything: "By putting kink in leg, see how much farther forward it brings sliding carrier," read the message on a crude drawing from El.

A water-stained note on the back of a Sohio receipt for an oil change survives: "Leo mentioned a split in profits on items we sell through him. Why not? A half a loaf of bread is better than none for both of us." Dick, who had written the suggestion in his looping cursive, favored paying the fee to keep Ferno's products in Leo Hodroff's Kelco catalog. El took a calculated look at the loaf, finding that Ferno would lose 10 cents each on Kelco's suggested pricing of cot conversions.

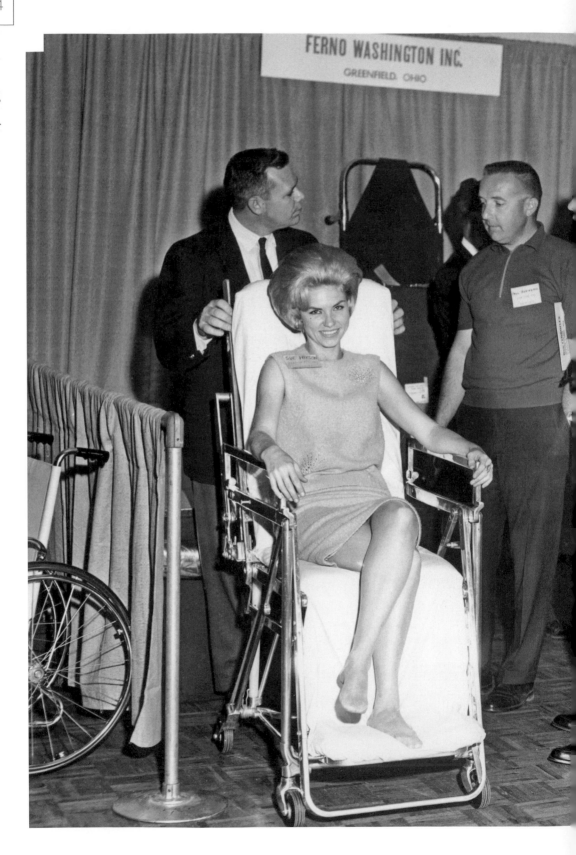

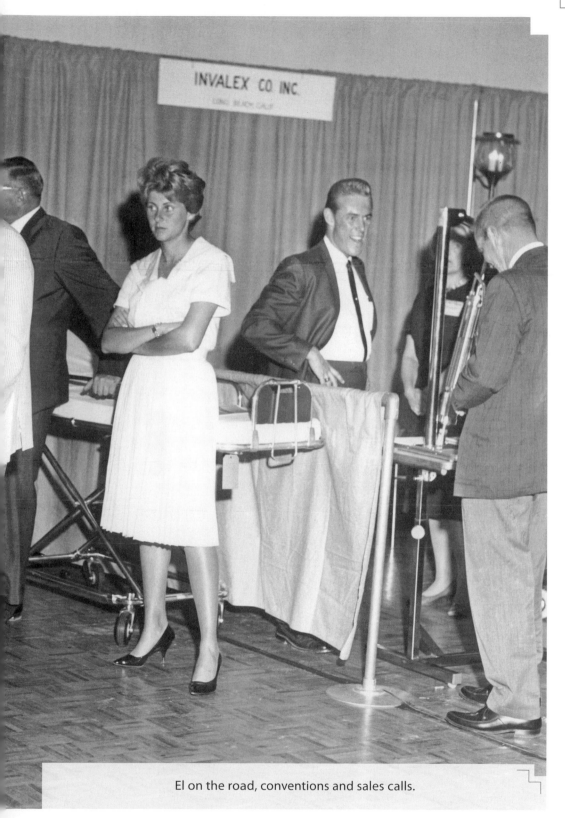

El on the road, conventions and sales calls.

In December of 1956, Ferno severed its agreement with Kelco and hired Howard Swink Advertising of Marion, Ohio, to overhaul the company's promotional materials, expand advertising and publish a colorful new catalog of its own, marketing aggressively to the mortuary and EMS businesses.

Swink also made connections with the press.

El sent a note to his partner on a scrap of stationery from the Jung Hotel in New Orleans, billed as the "South's largest air-conditioned 1200 rooms," clipped to a photo of a Ferno stretcher from the *Times-Picayune*. "The Front Page!" he crowed.

Swink's industrious clipping service sent an astonishing and sometimes bizarre array of Ferno products in the news. Marilyn Monroe was wheeled from the Los Angeles County Coroner's Office to Westwood Village Mortuary for final rites on a Ferno cot. A recovering burn victim was lifted into an ambulance by her prom date on a One-Man Cot. Rescue workers in Tucson were pictured pulling survivors from a plant explosion on the Scoop. A Mt. Everest climber with frostbite was taken down the mountain on a Scoop, then shown arriving at Dulles Airport on a Ferno Stretcher Chair. When Lt. Col. John Glenn Jr. fell during his Senate campaign, he was transported to the hospital on a Ferno cot.

As efficient media monitors scrutinized the nation's newspapers and magazines in search of Ferno products, El Bourgraf was just as intently scanning the horizon for bootleg cots and design poachers. He was fiercely protective of Ferno's grip on the market.

A prominent ad in a 1957 edition of *The Atlanta Journal-Constitution* warned, "Patent applications covering our One-Man Cots are now on file in the Patent Office. Other makers of similar cots are used and sold at the risk of appropriate court action." He hired patent attorney William Konold of the Cincinnati law firm of Wood, Herron & Evans, who not only pounced on infractions but at El's instruction began exploring the patent laws in other countries.

Ferno matured in stature and merchandise, burnishing its reputation.

Dave Haines remembered getting a call in 1967 from a representative of the Israeli government. "They wanted 10,000 stretchers. Now." Ferno's stretcher production then was about 500 or 600 a week. "We had maybe 200 in stock," El said. A hasty meeting was called over the weekend.

"We didn't have that kind of material or capacity," Dave said. But this was a serious request, followed by phone calls from Sen. Jacob Javits of New York, who helped round up materials from an aluminum mill in New Jersey." Future senator Howard Metzenbaum, a Cleveland businessman active in Jewish affairs, checked in with offers of help.

The following week, phone calls poured in from America's Jewish community:

"I've got semis if you need materials brought."

"I've got a plane."

The company continued normal daily production and at night everybody, even the office crews, returned to work on the stretchers. Women from the sewing room dashed out at 4:30, went home and fixed dinner for their families and came back. "We worked twenty-four hours a day, seven days a week," Dave said. "That's something I'll always remember. With that type of cooperation and participation you could do most anything. And we did."

Across the world, in June of 1967 Israel and the neighboring states of Egypt (then the United Arab Republic), Jordan and Syria fought what was to be known as the Six-Day War. By then, 6,000 stretchers had been shipped from Wilmington. "They took everything we made, and asked we stop production at that point," El said. "I will never forget the way our people stepped up."

Bernie Zoldak, naturally, was in the thick of the Israeli project, as well as everything else. He was El's financial right arm and now his left arm up to the shoulder, working on quality control and purchasing. Bernie was hired to relieve El, and others were hired to take some of the pressure off Bernie. Ferno was big. And getting bigger.

"We had ninety to ninety-five percent of the emergency and mortuary business," El said. The Bomgardners had moved to Florida and were selling oxygen supplies. Washington Mortuary Supply was hurting and their business was shrinking.

Still, El faced the same old problem: how to grow a company whose products didn't wear out and—not counting a once-in-a-lifetime run on stretchers—were not needed in great volume. "We would go into a town and sell a cot to the funeral home and the ambulance service there," El said. "And that was it for them for five, ten or twenty years."

El, Dick, and Bernie looked into compatible products. When 3M replaced the Thermofax copier, it was so big, it took two men to carry it. Ferno built a cart that could allow a single person to transport it. The first copy machine was a little smaller than a card table and weighed about 200 pounds. Like the vintage funeral cot, it took two salesmen to haul it into an office. The one-man SalesMaker was created. "It rolls on large rubber-tired wheels, slides over the edges of steep steps on nylon glides and the telescoping handle locks for easy pushing and pulling without bending your back or hitting your heels." A smaller version was pitched to schools and offices for moving cumbersome audio visual equipment, typewriters and furniture.

Another niche. But still a niche.

Dick was cautious. El was impatient. Innovation and modification continued, edging inexorably toward life-saving, rather than end-of-life handling. Along with the Model 22 Mortuary Cot and Model 86 Church Truck, in quick succession, Ferno-Washington introduced, the Model 28 Ferno-Flex chair cot, the Model 26 One-Man Roll-In Ambulance Cot, and Model 30 All-Level Cot. The Model 60 Full-Length Foldable Spine Board, an improved Model 23 Mortuary Cot with an extended wheelbase for larger bodies and the folding Model 102 Mortuary Table were on the drawing board.

Ferno-Washington had its own elaborate catalog and carefully honed mailing list, selling through 1,200 distributors. They were outgrowing their plant at Greenfield. And Dick Ferneau wanted out.

The Long Goodbye

When El Bourgraf talked about his partner, he smiled. Always. Sometimes shook his head a little. Fond? For sure. Baffled? Just a little.

"Richard was a very complex man," he'd say. Richard. Most everybody, from the guy polishing a caster fork to the Vice President of Something Important to the corporate lawyer, referred to the co-founder of the company as "Dick." Familiar. Comfortable. Casual. El's careful reference to his partner by his given name, and notes written to him addressed to "Henry," a long-standing joke between them, hint at a relationship that was not simple. Affectionate. Respectful. But complicated.

Writing to Burt Weil, Dick revealed his insecurities: "You, El and Leo Hodroff are the three most important persons in my life, and heaven only knows where I would be or what I would be doing had it not been for the three of you. I guess I am just a misfit. I don't know why I let the boat pass me by." Dick Ferneau said he admired what he called the "class" of the three men.

"You did not have a lot handed to you on a silver platter, nor did El. I remained a clod while you and El forged ahead in your learning, manners, religion and social life. I can only blame myself, for there was no one holding me from doing the same." Ironically, he laments his lack of education eloquently, in perfect grammar, with flawless penmanship.

In letters to confidants beginning in 1966 when Dick was in his late 40s, he signals his inclination to back away from the business: "I feel El will forge ahead better without a partner, for he is more than able to run that business or any business very efficiently. He has the ability and confidence and desire to be what he is, one fine guy and businessman. I have always been so proud of my association with him."

He wrote to Burt Weil, "I feel I am just putting my days back of me FAST. I can't enjoy what I have for the driven feeling I have had since I was fourteen years old." He complained that he was bored, had lost the "fire in the belly." As the workforce expanded, he was wistful for the days in the Staunton garage when he had one employee "who could make patterns and operate any kind of machine." Presumably without being told what to do. A genius at design and a master of assembly, Dick Ferneau liked being in the shop, but not as foreman. He'd rather fix something himself than tell somebody else how to do it.

A large health care company in Milwaukee flirted. No formal offer was made, but they floated some numbers. Dick's interest was piqued. El consulted Bill Gradison, an investment broker and banker he'd met in college working on Bob Taft's campaign. Gradison, who later served as a U.S. congressman for nearly two decades, warned him this would be exactly the wrong time to sell.

"Bill believed we could grow and increase the company's worth significantly," El said, "but I think this triggered Dick's desire to leave. He thought he wanted to spend his time fishing, and he talked about going to Las Vegas," El said. "Everybody tried to talk him out of it. Me especially."

Engineer, Burt Selig, who worked with Dick back in the Washington Court House days and was a consultant to Ferno, had a heart attack en route to work, wrecked his car and died, adding to Dick's melancholia.

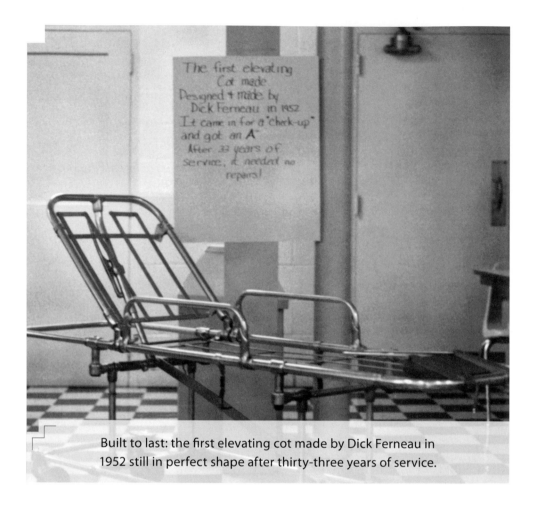

The first elevating
Cot made
Designed + made by
Dick Ferneau in 1952
It came in for a "check-up"
and got an "A"
After 33 years of
service, it needed no
repairs!

Built to last: the first elevating cot made by Dick Ferneau in
1952 still in perfect shape after thirty-three years of service.

After a phone call from Dick in early 1967 announcing he was selling his house, El implored him to take a year off. "Continue to draw your salary," he said. "I like to think after a year, you'll come back with some off-beat ideas that will mean more business and profits for both of us. Take off, goof off, get lost, get found, and get relaxed enough to come back."

Their mentor Burt Weil spoke to Dick, suggesting it might simply be a mid-life crisis, beseeching Dick to talk with Lucien Cohen, a highly regarded industrial psychologist in Cincinnati. "He has been called into consultation for years by firms with executives facing the same problems. Please, Dick, give him two hours of your life. Call him now!"

Burt Weil sent a copy of this letter to El with a handwritten note at the top: "If this works, and I think the chances are 1 in 100, I expect you to double my pickle allotment this Christmas."

Ever polite, Dick Ferneau thanked Weil for his suggestion, reiterating his determination and ending, naturally, with this note: "The third-level One-Man looks good with the new pattern work and castings." Privately, he complained to El that Burt wanted to send him to a "headshrinker." On an especially stressful day sorting out personnel and shipping problems, he followed with a note joking "maybe it's time I went to the man with the white coat and got a reading."

But he didn't.

An intense exchange began—letters, notes, and conversations. "I am completely satisfied with our association as it exists today," El insisted.

"In October of 1957, we sat in your kitchen and decided our personalities and abilities complimented each other, and I was willing to gamble on our combined efforts. So many things have happened. Every year has been different for different reasons, but I know I made the right decision then. We have achieved success and security," he wrote in a rambling letter in March of 1967.

"Corny as it sounds, we have done it as a team. Some of the happiest days of my life were the crazy ones when we worked from dawn to midnight trying to come up with the #30. We made some mistakes but we turned right around and went back to work and ended up with a good product. My whole point is that we have had some pretty good days as a result of problems and bucking heads to solve them. In the better than ten years we have worked together, I don't feel we have ever had an honest-to-goodness argument. Differences of opinion, YES. But never a down and out argument that tarnished our mutual respect or ability to work together," he continued.

"I cannot figure out how to replace our ability to share a crisis together, whether it be a competitive threat, a union threat or a meaningful decision. It goes back to the adage that management is lonely, the price of being the boss. Such things you can't share with a wife, or with someone that works for you. Even with Bernie, as good as he is. I'm sure you have the feeling that some things are off limits because he works for us. Sharing the loneliness, not having to spell out all the P's and Q's, not having to put up with general meaningless talk is one of the cornerstones and foundations of our business and success."

Dick's handwritten reply was to thank El for "the review of our history. Granted it has been a mixture of challenges. Glad it was with someone like you. This is no snap decision, but time is the most precious thing anyone has, and he never knows how much or little he has. Since I can remember, work has come first, and personal life where I could grab it."

Later that month, Dick wrote to El, proposing they look for a buyer, maybe pursue the Milwaukee suitors. "Things have rung the caution bell in the back of my head indicating perhaps our efforts wouldn't be as rewarding as they have been. I was in hopes you wouldn't want to press your luck either and would try to find an outfit that would be to our liking and interested in giving us top price. The time to sell, of course, is when you have something to sell. Or maybe," he wondered, "you might have someone to take my place."

El, persistently optimistic about Ferno's future and buoyed by advice from Gradison, told Dick Ferneau he'd rather go it alone. "I'm not looking for another partner. You just don't find the equal partner relationship you and I have enjoyed every time you try. It's just like I say about hiring a friend. I was lucky with Bernie, and I'll never test my luck again. If I lose you as a partner, I'm better off in the long run without a partner."

In early April on Ferno letterhead, El dispatched a typewritten proposal, saying he'd consulted outside advisers and experts. Which he cheerfully ignored. "I am relying on my own judgment and knowledge of how we have always dealt with each other." He'd been advised to establish a conservative value and not to make his best offer first. "I chose to see how much loot I could come up with, and relate it to the sense of security it would offer you. I felt this is really what you were interested in, and I hope I was not wrong. If I am, we can go back and start over."

Bernie Zoldak projected the company's total net worth as of June of 1967, estimating combined holdings in the business at $500,000. This was slightly higher than the offer tendered previously by the health care company and took into account El's confidence that the company would continue to grow, allowing Dick to participate in its success.

"I'm proposing a total payout to you of roughly $466,000," El wrote.

Zoldak, the much-beloved bean counter, worried that the cash demands of El's proposition would hamper the company's growth and pointed out gently that the offer assumed El's continued good health and untested ability to run the business alone. "It's just a shame that the combination that has been so successful can't continue," he said.

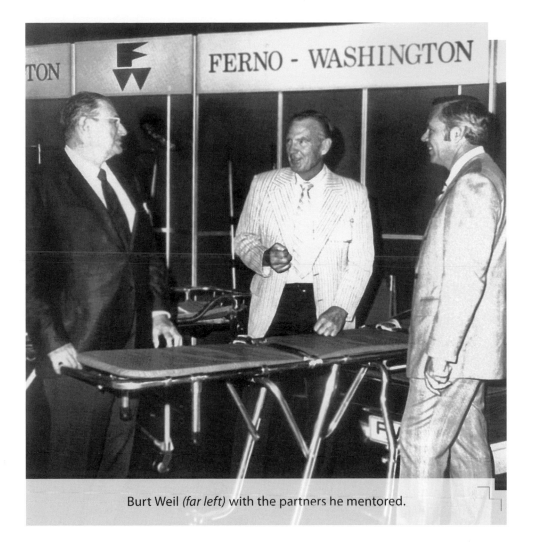

Burt Weil *(far left)* with the partners he mentored.

The document from El was straightforward and detailed, including cash plus installment payments over eight years, a retirement account, medical insurance and a recapture clause if the business was sold for a greater amount during the payout period. Pretty standard stuff, except that El's plan also outlined tax obligations for the seller and advice from a financial planner suggesting investment options. "Fully realize that I have stuck my nose where it shouldn't be," El wrote, "but I guess I did it from habit."

The letter was signed not Elroy Bourgraf, or even El. The signature at the bottom of the careful document spelling out the termination of this unusual and warm relationship was simply, Ish, the nickname used only by Dick Ferneau and Bernie Zoldak.

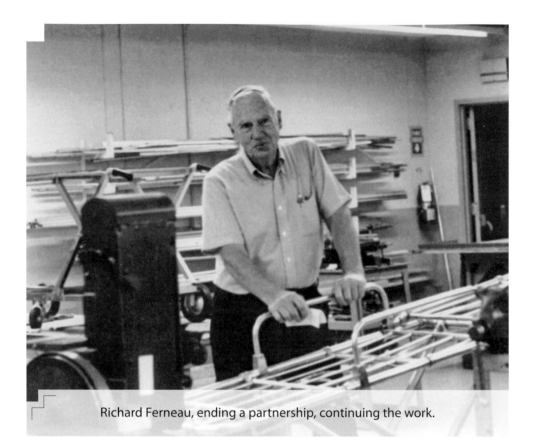

Richard Ferneau, ending a partnership, continuing the work.

Some modest back-and-forth with details and an agreement from Dick that he'd continue as a paid consultant preceded a blizzard of legal papers. And the inevitable personal letter: "Ish, I have a feeling of pride having you for a partner and not once did I feel like I was leaving you with more than you could carry. In any situation that I can be of assistance, I will be there, even as an outsider. It is still our baby, and I will help you raise it any time you may need me."

El dictated a memo to employees in February of 1968:

"After thirty years in the industry, Dick Ferneau has decided to get free from the day-to-day plant routine. You may have already noticed he is harder to pin down than ever. Dick will continue to be active in market research, new product development and help us in a consulting capacity." In a letter dated June 27, 1968, Richard H. Ferneau officially tendered his resignation. He had just turned 49. El Bourgraf was 37 years old.

Dick just faded away. No party. No cake. No speeches. Anything else would have been agony for him. Nobody saw him clear out his desk. There wasn't much to be cleared from his office—about a shoebox full. Most of his time at the company had been spent in the plant. He told Bernie Zoldak how to reach him in an emergency and then disappeared for two months. Then he "popped in just like always," El said. He just didn't stay as long or come as often. The precise mechanical diagrams and quirky letters continued for the next twenty years. In 1987 he officially retired, by then the owner of sixteen patents.

In 1990, the National Association of Emergency Medical Technicians awarded him its highest honor, the Rocco V. Morando Lifetime Achievement Award, noting, "Any EMT or paramedic who has moved a patient owes a debt of gratitude to Mr. Ferneau."

Dick Ferneau passed away in 2009 at the age of 90.

A note on a scrap of yellowed paper in an untidy file left behind by Ferno's most senior founder: "Keeping a business running successfully is like pushing a load of perishables uphill. When you tire of pushing and take your shoulder away, you must have another's shoulder to continue the push."

"...when a Ferno employee leaves those meetings, they know as much about what's going on in this company as management does. And it's created a culture that says, I don't work for Ferno—I am Ferno."

3

Moving Forward

Family Ties

Joseph George Bourgraf, named for his grandfathers, was born on his father's birthday in November of 1960 in Greenfield. When he was a boy, Joe shuttled between a city where his mother's family sold pickles and sauerkraut and a town where his father owned the biggest emergency equipment plant in the world. He was thoroughly comfortable in both places.

Busy and bright, Joe was adored by the Kunkels, who took their oldest grandchild to the family sour goods stand at Findlay Market in downtown Cincinnati Wednesdays, Fridays and Saturdays when he was little. "I loved being there, seeing the way they worked, the pride in their business," Joe said.

He darted between barrels of every kind of pickled vegetable, sweeping, cleaning, and making himself useful just as his mother had done.

"My mother and father didn't believe in baby sitters," Elaine Bourgraf said. "They took me with them. When I was a baby I'd take my nap in a crate filled with overcoats." And though she didn't know him yet, around that same time her husband-to-be was napping in a coffin just a few blocks away, also sharing a workday with his father, a casket vendor.

As a teenager, Elaine Kunkel would slide her elegant narrow feet into heavy wooden clogs, ordered from Holland and hand rubbed and waxed by her mother and aunts. Then she would climb into a vat of chopped raw cabbage and stomp, layer the vegetable with brine and stomp some more, beginning the fermentation that resulted in sauerkraut prized by discriminating Cincinnati housewives. Some days she'd wield the heavy four-foot paddle, turning pickles as they soaked, gossiping with the Spies girls who worked at their parents' cheese stand nearby.

"We talked about who we would marry and what we wanted to be," Elaine (who El nicknamed "Kunk") said. She was drawn to El from the moment she saw him. "He just seemed like a person who would never let me down. And he never has."

Marriages are strained in lots of ways. The for-richer-for-poorer, in-sickness-and-in-health vows don't begin to cover all that tests a couple over a lifetime. What happens, for instance, when it is their child who is sick? Really sick.

A beautiful baby with a nimbus of pale hair, Brian Bourgraf was born in September of 1963 with an oddly puckered abdomen. Prune Belly, it was called. Of

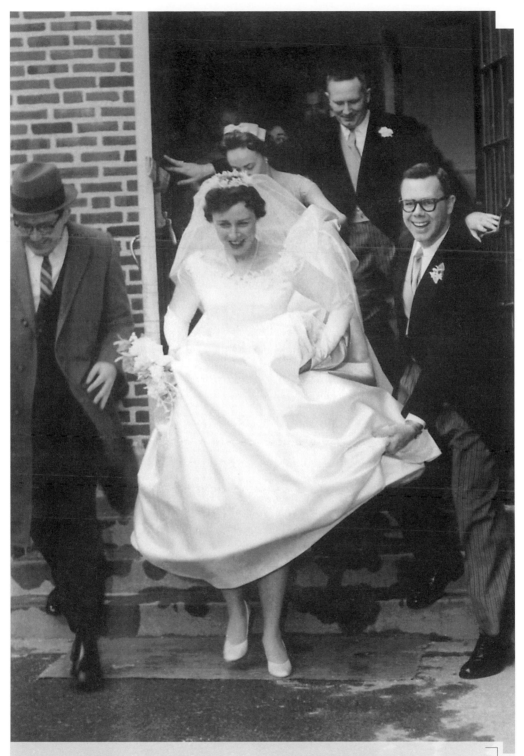

El and Elaine wed in February of 1960 on George Washington's birthday, chosen because the pickle stand would be closed for the holiday.

course, doctors used the condition's proper name, Eagle Barrett Syndrome, when they broke the news to his exhausted and worried parents. They told El and Elaine candidly that their second son's chances weren't good. A third of these children die before they reach the age of 2, and those who survive are gravely impaired. The syndrome is uncommon, occurring in approximately 1 in 30,000 to 40,000 live births. Boys make up about 95 percent of the cases. There's virtually no muscle in the walls of the abdomen, making it difficult if not impossible for the child to sit upright. Bladder and kidney problems. Urinary infections. Mobility uncertain. Possible bone damage. The list was long and the prognosis dire.

"El is a very level fellow," Elaine remembered. "He said, 'we can think it out.'"

El made phone calls, tapping his network of fraternity brothers, friends and business associates. A pioneer in pediatric nephrology, Dr. Clark West, was practicing at nearby Children's Hospital Medical Center in Cincinnati, and El wasted no time, pushing for an appointment. The busy physician "couldn't have been more helpful," El said. "I don't know what we'd have done without him."

El and Elaine took their baby to the highly regarded Cincinnati hospital, where Brian would spend two-and-a-half of the first four years of his life. When he was ten days old, an ileostomy bag was attached to his side, and a series of procedures—large and small—continued until he was able to leave the hospital. He would return many times in subsequent years for urgent care and remembers forbidden wheelchair races and nurses who slipped him treats. Sensitive and observant, he overheard them whispering about his condition, his chances in life and their conclusion—"we might as well let him enjoy what he wants."

The sound of his mother's clattering Bakelite bracelets would alert him that she was quick-stepping down the hallway, to read to him, to cheer him and, not incidentally, to learn how to care for him. She was also caring for a new baby, Elroy Edwin Bourgraf Jr.—El-B—who was born while his older brother was still in the hospital. "I managed to get home in time to see him born, but I was on the road a lot," El said. "Most of the care of the boys fell to Elaine. She kept everything going at home."

Responsibility for a chronically sick child and two more healthy ones, plus steering the tenuous early years of a family company was so profound that he knew it would have defeated anyone trying to carry on alone. It was not unusual for El to attend twenty-five or thirty conventions a year, then come back to a desk piled with paperwork, and people circling his office. Often, he brought clients home for a meal with a gracious hostess. His success with the business, he said, belongs to his wife "as much or more than anybody who was on the payroll."

Whenever Brian was allowed to come home, "He was a sick little guy most of the time, confined to his bed or a playpen," El said. Making a circle of her thumb and index finger, Elaine added, "His little legs were this big around." When Brian was four-and-a-half years old, he weighed seventeen pounds and had rickets. His body wasn't absorbing nutrients. He needed a new kidney.

In 1968, before he'd celebrated his fifth birthday, Brian had sixteen surgeries. The seventeenth would save his life. A double kidney transplant was performed at Children's Hospital by pediatric surgeons, Dr. Lester Martin and Dr. Louis Gonzales, using the organs of an infant with Brian's rare blood type who had died of hydrocephalus, or water on the brain.

After Brian's transplant, Joe said, "We always made sure of a relatively safe environment for him. He could do a lot of the things, and we had a lot of fun, but there were certain things that were just off limits. Tackle football was one of them, so we played flag football instead." Brian's younger brother, El-B, said, "I don't remember the actual transplant, but I remember he had to go back from time to time. They wouldn't allow me in the hospital because I was so young, so I stood outside with Dad or Mom with a walkie-talkie. I could see him up there in the window."

The Bourgrafs were advised that a school with a Montessori program was Brian's best chance to catch up with his age group. They also felt tethered to Cincinnati by its proximity to his doctors. Brian and his brothers all were enrolled at Summit Country Day School on the east side of Cincinnati, and the Bourgrafs rented an apartment at the Regency, a toney high-rise building a few blocks away, returning to Greenfield on weekends and during the summer. El commuted to Greenfield during the week on a B&O commuter train, now defunct.

Brian skied, played soccer and swam—all with a sunny disregard for the ordinary, hopping in the pool with the swim team wearing a tee-shirt over his patchwork of scars and his ostomy bag. Once at a meet, some fool hollered, "Take your shirt off," playing to the crowd.

And Brian said, "You really don't want me to do that." And then he dove in the pool, because he heard the gun.

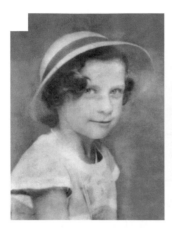
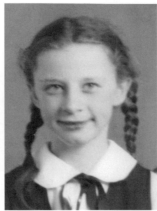
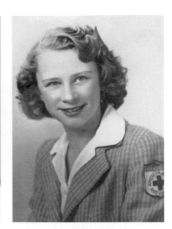

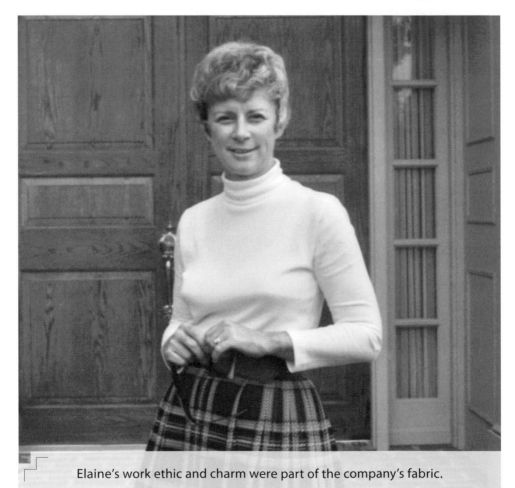

Elaine's work ethic and charm were part of the company's fabric.

Eventually, the family gave up the weekend commute to Greenfield and moved to a house in Indian Hill, a prosperous suburb just outside Cincinnati. Interior decorator for the Bourgrafs was Sarah Aronoff Weil, whom Burt married after his wife Olga's death from cancer in 1963. The house, while beautifully furnished, is comfortably, proudly a family home. Just off the sun room, a gallery of photos captures milestones of this family's life and also its modest beginnings. Among formal wedding and self-conscious school portraits are snapshots of Elaine posing on an ambulance cart, El barbecuing at a company picnic in a chef's hat, and the boys at summer camp.

Visitors descending the basement stairs find themselves entering a remarkably authentic scene from the old Findlay Market. A dramatically lighted wall mural of the family mingling with a crowd outside the Kunkel stand merges seamlessly onto real cobblestones and street details retrieved from the Over-the-Rhine neighborhood—an old mailbox, a fire hydrant, a telephone pole, a sewer vent, drain pipes, signs. It's so well done that it feels a little like a movie back lot or a skillfully painted stage set. You wouldn't really be surprised if Joseph Kunkel handed you a pickle. Furnishings include kegs, a cabbage cutter, a door from a wooden ice box, a scale and two pairs of wooden shoes—relics of the Kunkel business.

Elaine pointed to a portrait, repeating her grandmother's favorite claim, "I wear neither paint, nor powder. And the figure is all me own," delivering this line gleefully, with a credible Irish lilt. The wedding photograph captures Elaine's lovely and lively Irish grandmother on the day she joined the German immigrant family and became, by default, a sour goods maker and vendor. Another saying familiar to the Bourgraf boys was, "If you were a Kunkel, you were in the pickle business."

And Joe, Brian, and El-B would find out, in turn, and over sometimes turbulent years, whether being in the Bourgraf family meant that you were in the cot business.

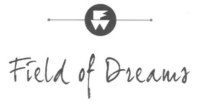

Field of Dreams

As Sarah Weil put the finishing touches on crown moldings and embossed wallpaper in the living room of the Bourgrafs' new home in suburban Cincinnati, El Bourgraf was absorbed in another move.

When Dick Ferneau and El bought the welding school property in Greenfield, it was too big. Before long, it was too small. At first, they leased half the space to a printing company. Then, they not only needed the rest of the building but

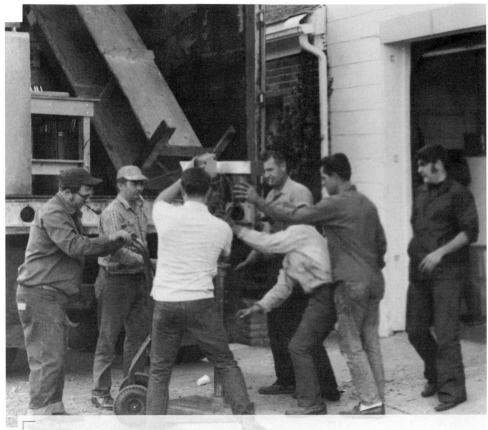

Leaving Greenfield for Wilmington.

the company's order processing operation was squeezed into a little gray-shingled house nearby. They picked up storage space in a garage and an abandoned barn, and a new subsidiary for research and development, Dielco, was housed in a small white cinder-block building in back. About forty feet wide and seventy feet long, it had the modest distinction of having its own restroom, which suffered chronic plumbing problems until the source of trouble was discovered—an alcoholic electrician using the toilet to chill his beer.

The idea for Dielco (a combination of Dick's and El's names) was to remove creation from manufacturing, with separate personnel and machinery, so that nobody had to stop work as a prototype was created and that parts were not cannibalized. A first draftsman—Dick called him a "draw-er"—was hired.

By the late 1960s, Ferno had nearly seventy people working in administration, sales, production and R&D in Greenfield and another thirty at the plant in

Washington Court House. There was no end in sight. El was having fun. Bernie was in charge at the office and El was "getting to do more of what I like to do, talking to customers." And listening, of course. Funeral directors didn't want to be in the ambulance business, but there were plenty of emergency-tested veterans returning from Korea and Vietnam wars who did. "These guys were great prospects for EMS and fire departments, changing the delivery of the emergency medicine landscape." El was spending a lot of his time getting to know this burgeoning market.

The new product line for the industrial safety and rescue market included the Basket Stretcher in "international orange, which meets military, mine and quarry, industrial requirements." It was selling like crazy. Orders were piling up and they were running out of storage. Even after he sold his share of Ferno, Dick was still a significant presence, working on new designs, floating in and out, staying in touch. He and El talked about the prospect of moving operations. Dick had the jitters, worried that a new building would be too expensive.

"I could never have gotten the company to its present stage," Dick wrote to El. "But I fear letting any weakness sneak up on it that would sap it from being strong, so that a union or competition could ever chip away at it."

Bernie Zoldak, cautious in his own way, believed the company would not only be stronger but more efficient if everything was under one roof. He suggested El take a look at nearby Wilmington's abandoned Air Force base. The town was reeling from the recent closing of the military installation.

Most of the drama revolved around 1,432 acres, which began in 1929 as a modest airport at the southeast edge of town. The original airstrip and single hangar morphed into the Clinton County Air Force Base, used by the U.S. Department of Defense as a Strategic Air Command refueling facility and for Special Ops training, preparing gunship crews for Vietnam. When the Department of Defense closed the base in 1971, more than 300 civilian jobs and an annual payroll of $9 million evaporated.

"We thought the world was going to come to an end," Wilmington banker, Robert Olinger, told the local newspaper. A Columbus *Dispatch* reporter wrote: "A tattered American flag graces the base administration building and waves lazily at half mast—an ironic salute to the death of the once busy facility."

Wilmington *News-Journal* editor Tom Hunter's account was vivid and anguished: "Nostalgia, really, has no place here. We want to be realistic. We don't want emptiness and silence. We want those gates to be unlocked. Rows and rows of vacant buildings that once housed the operations of some 2,500 human beings squat in abandonment, their sightless windows reflecting the will of the Department of Defense."

All was not lost. Financial disasters, unlike natural ones, leave intact buildings in their wake. The government dispatched a man, who said, "My orders are to pickle the property." This meant shutting off water, draining the lines, making sure that weather would not damage the structures.

Elroy Bourgraf was first to take a chance on one of the pickled buildings, and by July of 1972, he'd unlocked the gates and his company was up and running in spacious new quarters.

Things had moved fast after El picked out the building he wanted there. Mack Tool Company in Sabina put in a low-ball offer for the same space. El outbid them and cut a deal with Wilmington's Community Improvement Corporation (CIC), which still needed the title to the base. Federal officials, who weren't interested in being landlords or developers, told the CIC they'd float a loan at a seven percent interest rate if the CIC could come up with a down payment.

The city fathers rallied. Two local banks were persuaded to float short-term loans of $100,000 each, issuing checks to the CIC committee who traveled to Chicago, handed the checks over to the feds and signed a note for another $1 million. Then they turned right around and went back to Wilmington, where El waited with a check for $200,000 to pay off the banks.

"All that was accomplished in thirty-six hours," El said.

The *News-Journal* announced in jumbo type: FIRST INDUSTRIAL TENANT AT FORMER CLINTON COUNTY AIR FORCE BASE and followed with a twenty-two-page special section, reporting that the Ferno-Washington company carried 195 on its payroll and would use 800 gallons of paint and 680 square yards of carpeting on the renovation. Ads from Wilmington's merchants welcomed their new neighbor, and U.S. Secretary of Defense Melvin Laird traveled to the air base he'd closed and told the crowd of about 300, "As we turned the security of Vietnam over to the people of Vietnam, we had to make one million civil service reductions."

Well, yes, people there were familiar with the concept.

The space was good, but besides paint and new carpet, the building needed a new facade, landscaping, interior remodeling, and a new heating, ventilation, and air conditioning system. "When people used to talk about sweatshops," El said,

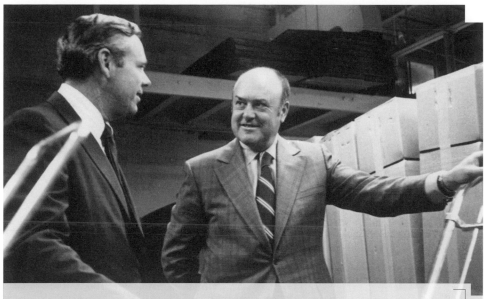

U.S. Secretary of Defense Melvin Laird traveled to the air base he'd closed to welcome El as the first new tenant.

"they meant real sweat. I think we were one of the first factories with central air. It was expensive, but the AC turned out to be a plus when we were hiring new people for the shop."

As work began on the renovation, El met with employees, reassuring them that their jobs were safe but some might have a longer commute to the new plant—which was twenty-two miles from Washington Courthouse and twenty-six from Greenfield. "We had people in maybe a fifty-mile circle, well over into Adams County, around Chillicothe, and a lot of those people continued to commute all the way to Wilmington," El said, "some driving sixty or seventy miles a day, each direction, until they retired."

Ferno also trolled the Wilmington area for new hires. "We were interested in keeping a stable workforce in the community and working with the other industries, so we didn't pilfer employees from each other. We tried to offer jobs to people who didn't have jobs, rather than steal them from one another," El said. Ferno also made jobs available to Wilmington folks who had found work in Cincinnati and Dayton after the Air Force left. "It was a very fertile source for talent."

Typically, when moving day arrived, El and Bernie rolled up their sleeves and gathered their employees. "We figured we'd just take all our guys, get some trucks

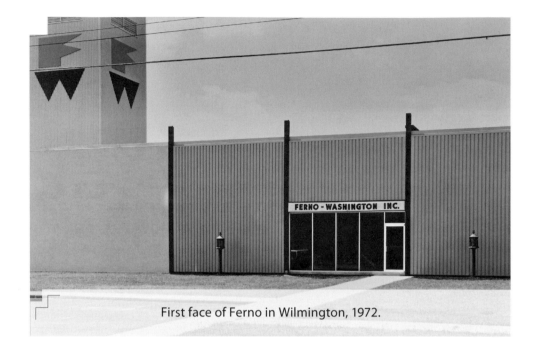

First face of Ferno in Wilmington, 1972.

and load up," El recalled. "Everybody moved their own department so when it got to Wilmington, they could put it where it belonged. We moved in two days. More or less."

They'd done a lot of work in advance—plotting the building layout on paper, measuring equipment and space, noting where they wanted the lathes, the drill presses, mills and benches. They marked up the floors with equipment locations and electrical diagrams. Semi-trucks showed up in Greenfield at 5 a.m. and were loaded and on the road by noon. Waiting in Wilmington was a crew ready to put everything back together. All the drill presses and most of the lathes were up and running the same day in Wilmington.

Long-time employee Irvin Pollock was perched atop a forklift that morning, hefting huge turret lathes and spindle drill presses to a flatbed semi. When he arrived in Wilmington and saw the square white tower, he had another of his "bright ideas." That tower, tall enough to dangle a parachute from the top and dry it with blasts of hot air, was solid and Ferno had no use for it.

"Before we moved," Irv said, "they said it was going to cost several thousands of dollars to get that taken down, to level it, and I told Bernie, I said, 'Well, why don't you just put FW on there?' and he said, 'That's a good idea,' so it's still there, and it has FW on it."

Irvin, who worked at every Ferno location, including Washington Court House, during his nearly forty-eight years with the company, said the thing he didn't mind leaving behind at Greenfield was the heat. The only relief from the hot air generated by busy machines was big fans and cold drinks. "It was hotter than blue blazes in the summer. They'd go down to Pierce's Restaurant for big kettles of lemonade and push a cart through the shop. Ice cold lemonade." He smacked his lips.

Thinking back to his first stifling day at Ferno-Washington, Irvin remembered Bert Selig, who'd worked with Dick Ferneau to design the first hospital-bed-height cot. Bert saw the youngster leaning against a workbench, gulping a nickel bottle of pop. There was no caste system at Ferno. Not then. Not now.

"Hi, Sonny," he said. "Come over here and let me show you what I'm working on."

Almost overnight, the air conditioning, the vending machines, and everybody was under one roof. Dielco was now just an area, squared off, with the floor painted blue. The grinding room was making its familiar racket, and Bernie Zoldak had hung his jacket over the back of his chair and put his files neatly in order. El's secretary, Millie Head, was at her desk, which no longer contained the boss's cigarettes. Bob Mottie was assembling a #30 all-level cot and Larry Johnson was packing up a Scoop for shipping.

El's challenge was to make sure the spirit that brought these people together to build a walker for a little girl and a mountain of stretchers for Israel would also survive the move to new quarters and be up and running the same day.

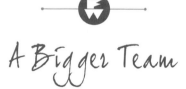

A Bigger Team

As the company grew, El delegated. He was good at that, good at finding talent, and good at riding along with them before he took off the training wheels.

Gary Hiles met El when he was nine years old, mowing the grass at the Bourgraf house in Greenfield. Later, he was their paperboy, delivering the *Cincinnati Post* in the afternoon. El could spot work ethic when he saw it and arranged for the neighbor kid to work at his plant during the summer.

"I worked in the manufacturing area." Gary said. "When I went to UC's community college, for the first two years I worked for Elroy in the morning, did all

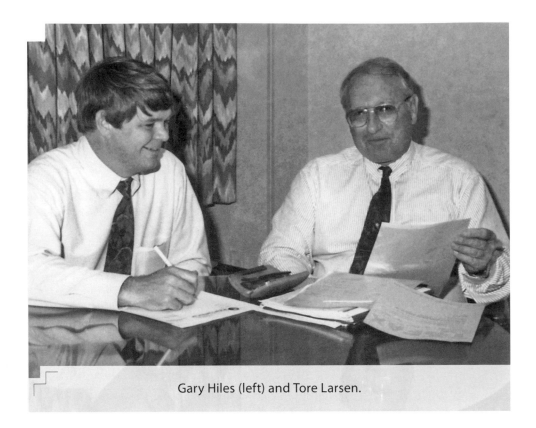

Gary Hiles (left) and Tore Larsen.

odd job-type things, gofer-type work, and then went to school at night. I finished the last two years down on the campus, down in Cincinnati." After graduation in 1972, he set about finding a job, looking around Cincinnati. One day, he stopped off at the plant in Wilmington. "Just to say hello to El. I hadn't had a chance to see him for a while."

Affable as ever, the president and CEO of the company dropped everything to show off the new place. During the tour, Gary told El he'd been interviewing for jobs and had a couple of prospects. "So he calls my mom—because back in those days, you don't have cell phones—and says, 'Have Gary give me a call, I may have something for him for a while, for a short period of time.' So that's what I did, I gave him a call."

At first, new college graduate Gary Hiles counted cots and casters, taking inventory the old-fashioned way, before bar codes and scanning wands, marking time until he heard back from one of his real job prospects. Three months later, El offered him a job in Customer Service. "Elroy offered me a job on Wednesday, and then the other two companies I was interviewing for offered me a job on Thursday and Friday of the same week. So I didn't have a job, and then I had three jobs in one week."

He chose to stick with Ferno. And with El.

"He made absolutely no promises in the beginning, and I worked in the Customer Service area until '74," Gary said. "Then Elroy decided he wanted to cut down a little more of his domestic travel and get more involved internationally. He asked me if I'd be willing to travel domestically for him, to meet all the dealers, go to all the trade shows. I mean, he said, 'You want to go to Omaha, Nebraska? I said, 'El, I've never been to Omaha.' So we went to the American Ambulance Association (AAA) Convention, me for the first time."

That was in September of 1974. A month later, El sent Gary to Chicago to the National Safety Congress, a very big deal. "I'll show you how to set up the exhibition and you're going to be there," El told Gary.

"We were sitting in Chicago at the old Drake Hotel downtown, after the show. Elroy always gives you what I call life lessons, ways you can be successful in how you live your life. That evening, what he said was, 'if you never lie, then you never have to remember what you say.' And that stuck with me, you know, for years and years and years, and I still use that phrase a lot. Because that's the way I've kind of run my life since he said it, because that means a lot. It says a lot. And that's the way I run the International Department here. And when I did domestic things, that's the way I ran that department as well. It's a deep thought, if you think about it."

Once, Gary said, the boss told him something else he'd never forget. "I'll walk you to the mountain, and you have the choice. If you're afraid, you can walk around it. You won't see much. But if you want to walk to the top of it—and I'll help you—then you'll see some tremendous scenery."

Gary made the choice to climb.

The 1970s were a controlled whirl of motion at the top. El was adjusting to life without a partner. A bigger factory and more people meant more pressure to find products and customers to keep them all busy. He parceled out responsibility, brass rings on an administrative carousel that was picking up speed.

Gary Hiles was officially Field Sales Representative. Dale Hinman, who'd worked on Ferno business at Swink Advertising, joined Ferno as advertising manager and later headed up purchasing. Hinman, another Army vet, had a business degree from the University of Dayton and had been advertising manager for Bryant Air Conditioning in Indianapolis. Bernie Zoldak had moved up from office manager and purchasing agent to treasurer to the newly created position of executive vice president.

Ohio State University graduate Don Hindes, who started as sales manager for American Pad and Textile Co. in Greenfield, was named director of marketing and, later, vice president of corporate development. Washington Mortuary alum and University of Cincinnati graduate, Robert Miller, was production coordinator, then credit manager. Robert Dunn, director of engineering, had worked his way up from foreman of the Greenfield plant.

Bob Ginter, a Morehead State University grad, was tapped as head of personnel in 1977. Two things stick in his mind about his first meeting with the CEO. "Boy, is he big," Ginter thought. Then the big man started talking about the company, the people who worked with him. That was the second thing Bob will always remember.

"You could hear in his voice, the inflection in his voice—he was so excited, and he believed so strongly in where he was taking Ferno."

"You can have the most modern buildings that architects could build," El told Ginter. "You can have the most modern machinery that's on the market. You can have the best technology that's available. And you can have all the product innovation that's the latest and greatest. But if you don't have the people, and you don't have the loyalty of the people, you can't do anything."

Over the next thirty-five years, Ginter would have plenty of chances to see whether El Bourgraf meant what he said at that job interview. He had to listen carefully. Ferno didn't always do things by the book. Chemistry trumped the book every time. And family.

His assignment, he was told by management, was to up the ante on the education and skill level of the workforce. Bernie Zoldak told him, "We'll do a lot of that with training, but when we interview people, just make sure that they have some experience. And let's make sure they at least have a high school education."

Three days after that speech, Bernie buttonholed the new personnel director about an applicant. "I think we should hire him," Zoldak said.

Ginter pointed that the young man not only didn't have any experience, he had quit school after the eighth grade.

"Well, I know," his boss replied, "but his mom works here, and his dad works here, and his brother worked here before he went on to a better job. And they're all good people. I think we just go ahead and hire him."

Ginter said, "I was thinking, uh-oh, what have I gotten myself into?" He said he found out that Ferno hired people "based upon our thoughts of their ability to do the job."

During El's tenure as board president at Wilmington College, he handed out learning certificates to inmates at nearby Lebanon Correctional Institute. And he hired some of them.

"I had the opportunity to meet their families and see what a difference it could make to a whole lot of people if they got a chance to work, to prove themselves. Plus I had a chance to see what kind of support they had." El was willing to make that leap of faith. "Probably not very businesslike," the CEO said. Just like those one-of-a-kind projects where the bill "got lost." Maybe not very businesslike but certainly very El-like.

Considering Elroy Bourgraf's military leadership experiences—commanding ROTC drills and, later, as an Army lieutenant in Germany—his business style over the years has been remarkably collegial, perhaps a result of also leading a fraternity house full of opinionated and easily distracted undergraduates. Perhaps a natural blend of leadership and his talent for making a sale.

The rewards of El Bourgraf's brand of employee management, Bob Ginter said, are substantial and, in the crunch, very good business. "One time we had a customer from Canada who had to have an order, and it had to be done quickly— one of those moment's-notice type things. We asked for volunteers and got them. We worked all night long. And when they came down the next morning, that order was ready to go. I ran from here to Dayton to the plater's to get parts plated. We'd get ten parts made, I'd run them up to Dayton, pick up the parts they'd just plated, run them back. All night long. And it was management and production working together to get the thing done."

Another time, a holiday weekend, there was a problem with a shipment, desperately and immediately needed by a customer. "We called our people together. Now, they got off at 3:30 in the afternoon. At 3:00, we called those people and we said, look, here's the situation—here's the customer, here's what's happened. We need some people to work tomorrow, Saturday, on a holiday week.

If you don't want to, we understand. But we'd sure appreciate it. We had more people than we needed."

At first, he was a little surprised by the open, really open, communication. "We have an open-door policy. And you say, well, yes, everybody has an open-door policy. But we really do have an open-door, and an open-book policy. We have those group meetings once every quarter where everybody gets together. We talk. We talk about what's going on that's good, we talk about what's going on that's bad. We talk about how much money each entity of Ferno has made, how much profit they've made. We talk about quality problems.

"When a person—when a Ferno employee leaves those meetings, they know as much about what's going on in this company as management does. And it's created a culture that says, I don't work for Ferno—I am Ferno."

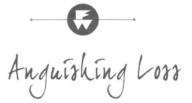

Anguishing Loss

Mary Lou Zoldak remembered the first time she saw Greenfield on a trip to visit their old friend, El. A bright winter day, made brighter by the pristine blanket of new snow. "Beautiful, a picture postcard of a small town." As she and Bernie drove down the main drag, they stopped, turned to each other and roared with laughter. Propped against a tree was a hand-lettered sign with an arrow: "Bern, I live here." Classic El.

Fresh off the troop ship from Germany, the couple was headed for Oklahoma. The plan was still for Bernie to put in his twenty years as a career Army officer. After the USS Randall voyage from Bremerhaven to New York, Mary Lou was not so sure. "I pictured life as an Army wife as a series of these trips. I told Bernie if he ever put me on a ship again, I'd kill him."

They left Greenfield, promising to stay in touch. And they did. When El had a chance to visit them at the base in Oklahoma, he offered Bernie a job at his company. "El gave us some time to think about it. It was a big decision, because the Army life had been our plan, but both of us had a lot of faith in El. He just exuded success. And I liked the idea of putting down roots in that pretty little Ohio town."

But she told her husband that it was strictly up to him. "I'm the tail on your kite, I used to say. We just did it and didn't analyze. In those days, we didn't sweat the details. I think back and I can't believe how we made it work."

When they moved to Greenfield, Mary Lou discovered it wasn't easy to meet people. "We didn't have any kids in school. Finally, we were so desperate we joined a square dancing group. Neither of us had ever square danced but we wanted to make friends." Soon a female ally arrived, one who became a friend for life.

Bernie Zoldak,
a fortunate connection.

"After El and Elaine got married, Elaine started a newcomers club. She also started a pre-school group, the Merry-Go-Rounders. It was a play group. Elaine thought kids just didn't get to see enough of the world. We'd take field trips to the fire station, to the air base in Wilmington. She was just like El, a go-getter, too. They made a good couple."

Bernie threw himself headlong into the new job. "Bernie liked his job right away. Boy, did he ever," Mary Lou said. "He loved setting up things at a new company. Those boys—El and Bern and Dick—worked a lot of hours." Bernie came home for lunch every day. "I loved that, the break in my lonely day. On Fridays, he was always in a hurry because he had to rush to the bank and make a deposit so the payroll checks would be good that afternoon."

The Zoldaks built a house after six years in Greenfield, big, with four bedrooms for their growing family—two daughters and a son. Fifty years later, El remembered the telephone number at this house. "I should. I must have called that number a thousand times." When the company moved to Wilmington, the Zoldaks stayed put in Greenfield. Bernie went on to serve as president of the Greenfield Rotary Club there, as well as two terms on the city council and a member of the hospital board of trustees.

Young and energetic, they knew, she said, all of them, including the wives that they were building something lasting, something important. One evening, she remembers dinner at Snow Hill Country Club, just outside Wilmington. Don and Jane Hindes, El and Elaine, Dick and Shirley Ferneau, and Bernie and Mary Lou lingered over dinner and talked. "We knew how rare this was, everybody pulling together, pulling for something. We felt so lucky."

The momentum continued with new products and upgraded equipment, including a state-of-the-art computer system. The Model 29, a roll-in multilevel cot for higher ambulances was introduced, along with the Model 50 combination transporter and Model 150 lift-off top for the international market. Models 35A and 35B roll-in cots went into production. The company pressed forward, continuing to improve patient care and safer, easier operation by attendants, building on the back-saving, labor-saving qualities of the Model 30 and the Model 26.

"I saw Ferno become a state-of-the-art corporation," Bob Ginter said. "When I started, we had a few emergency products, a few mortuary products, some sales cart products, so on and so forth. Any formal systems, they were just starting. I've seen it grow over the years and get better over the years. We've improved this, we've tweaked this, we've tweaked that. Now, I think we're a state of the art corporation, worldwide. I think we're state-of-the-art in employee talent, facilities, machinery, products. I've seen it come a long way."

Bernie was in charge of getting the new computer system up and running. Mary Lou thought that might be why he seemed so tired. The bounce had gone out of his step. When he went for a dental checkup, his dentist said he didn't like the looks of a redness in Bernie's throat. "It didn't hurt and he didn't have trouble swallowing or anything, but Bernie went to a doctor in Wilmington and had it biopsied."

They had been told it was epithelioma, which is often benign. She remembered that day clearly. "It was December 10, 1976. Bern came home early that day from work, and I can still see the look in his eyes. Bless his heart, he came home to tell me."

It's cancer, he told her. He was only 42 years old. He would beat it, he said.

Radiation treatments in Columbus started right away. Dick Ferneau drove them. The impossible-to-pigeonhole inventor and loner put aside his drafting pencils and became their chauffeur. The radiation wasn't working, and El put them in touch with doctors in Cincinnati, who told them the disease was an aggressive lymphoma and started him on chemotherapy. During all this time, Bernie continued going to his office in Wilmington, cheerful and effective. Optimistic.

The new treatments didn't work. "Tumors just kept popping up everywhere." Still, Bernie insisted on going to work. Mary Lou went with him "so he wouldn't stay all day." He lost his hair, and Dick Ferneau insisted he get a wig and took him shopping. He thought it might make Bern feel better.

Doctors recommended an experimental drug, which meant he had to stay at Cincinnati's Holmes Hospital during treatments. The Ferno family prayed and traded anxious condition updates. Six weeks in the hospital. They knew Bernie's condition was grave. El brought work to Bernie while he was in the hospital to keep him interested, to buck him up. "I don't know what I'd have done without El and Elaine," Mary Lou said. "I stayed at their house a lot." And, of course, Dick drove her back and forth. "He was at our beck and call."

A.B. "Bernie" Zoldak, still greatly mourned, died April 21, 1978.

If you look globally at our industry, there's not one innovative thought that wasn't generated by Ferno...Elroy never copied anything—he just improved it. Ferno is a brand that reflects the man.

4

Branching Out

Getting Back on Track

Toward the end of the 1970s, the momentum at Ferno-Washington sputtered. "I was in neutral," El said. Losing Bernie Zoldak was a tremendous setback. He was more than just an executive vice-president and treasurer. He was a confidant, a friend, and a talented insider. Neutral, however, was not El's customary speed. He shouldered his grief, his disappointment in what might have been, and hit the gas pedal. Forward. Drive.

El searched for someone to take over the reins inside the plant. Dave Haines took up the slack in the shop when El was on the road. Marketing director Don Hindes, who'd been with the company since the early days, was still in place. Bob Ginter was given more responsibility. Gary Hiles was succeeding beyond even El's high expectations.

A widow named Grace Rose, who'd been trained by Bernie in Greenfield, quietly pushed the paperwork through the system, writing checks, keeping the books. "A stalwart," El says, "completely trustworthy and detail oriented." The Ferno family rallied, continuing to do the jobs they'd been hired to do. A very large world beckoned, nudging El for attention, like this one on the letterhead of New South Wales Ambulance Transport:

"Our stretcher arrived this morning. Words cannot express our very sincere appreciation for a beautiful product. I have been in the ambulance service for thirty-one years, and I have never seen one to equal it. Now, we may have a problem with further imports. There is a firm who makes one of these stretchers in this country but nowhere near the product that yours is. Customs has come up with the bright idea that if an ambulance service can obtain a similar product in this country and we import a stretcher, then we must pay import duties.

"At present, we are having a ding dong go with customs, explaining that your product is better. PLEASE NOTE: Whatever happens, there will still be a definite order for two more stretchers and two more mattresses, even if we have to pay import duty."

El was getting clear signals that Ferno products were valued beyond U.S. borders, that customers were willing to pay a premium price for quality and innovation, and this one, at least, was even willing to have a "ding dong go" with his own government.

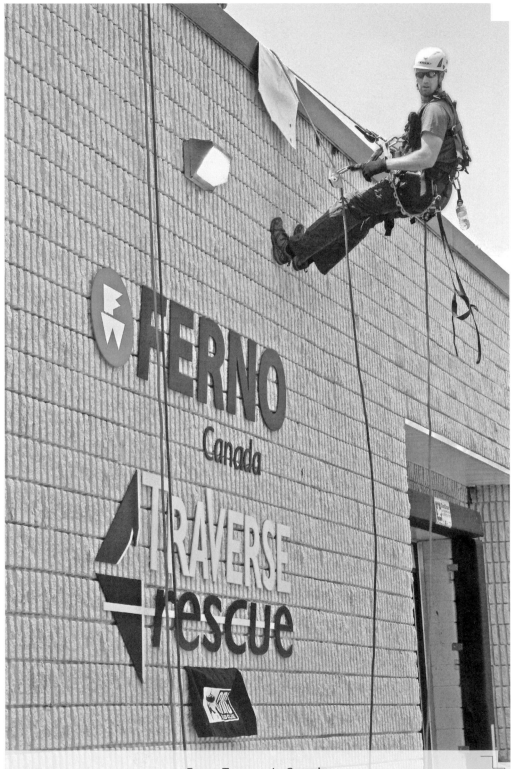

Ferno Traverse in Canada.

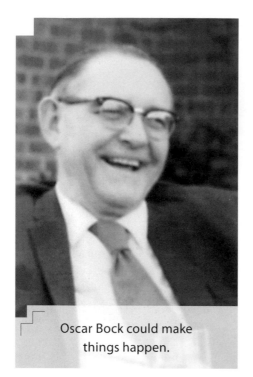

Oscar Bock could make
things happen.

Ferno's foreign business had been handled since the 1960s by a classy but casual outside sales representative. Rudy Fleck, who had been Studebaker's international sales manager before the auto company folded, wasn't exactly knocking on doors and making cold calls. Or even making phone calls. He more or less filled the orders, if they came in.

"He never traveled," El said. Rudy managed everything by Telex and mail from an office in South Bend, Ind. "He never touched a product and rarely touched a telephone. He had a lot of contacts from his years with Studebaker, and he was very well liked. A gentleman from the word go. A good listener. He really got me to appreciate that you had to adjust your sales approach to the culture of the country and not force American ways." If somebody in England or France or Germany wanted an American product, they'd remember Rudy and ask him to find the manufacturer and see if they could do business. He also had a few agents abroad, who sent orders his way.

"International shipping was a mystery to small companies." El said. "And kind of a pain. It might be six months from order to delivery."

Rudy Fleck's own company, Global Traders, had begun specializing in medical equipment and supplies. "International customers came to us." El said. "Somebody would see our literature and get in touch with him. We were glad to let Rudy handle it."

Rudy retired and sold the business to one of his field agents, Oscar Bock, his polar opposite in many ways. Bombastic and pear shaped, if the pear had been balanced upright by size fourteen shoes, Oscar "made some things happen," El remembered, traveling to foreign conventions and making connections to be cultivated by somebody else. Gary Hiles came to be the "somebody else," and an administrative team back in Wilmington put procedures in place to track orders, shipments, bills of lading, and receivables. After a couple of years of gradual transition, "We took over the business ourselves."

It had become increasingly clear that the complexities of international shipping were worth sorting out. And it would take Ferno's front-burner attention to do it.

During Rudy's time with Ferno, he had made a key connection. "Rudy Fleck found Appleyard and Les Harris," El said.

Leslie Harris, managing director of Appleyard Coach Builders in Bradford, England, often outfitted his company's ambulances with Ferno products bought

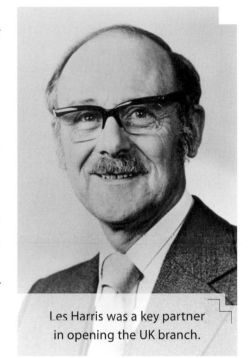

Les Harris was a key partner in opening the UK branch.

through Rudy Fleck. Appleyard relocated, reorganized, and pronounced Les Harris at the age of 50 "redundant," as his very British son, Peter, put it.

As many good things in life do, "it started with a little bit of adversity," Peter Harris said. Les examined his options. He could remain in the ambulance-building trade or, he thought, he might "sell the Ferno products in a dedicated company, rather than just fit them *ad hoc* into the occasional ambulance."

Les had met El previously, liked him and believed the Ferno chief would listen. He set up a meeting, proposing exclusive rights to distribution of Ferno products in his country. "My father outlined the idea, and Elroy could see potential in this," Peter said. Re-energized, Les Harris located a small warehouse in nearby Wyke and sold a variety of products, not all of them from Ferno. Some had to be assembled and, as Peter said, "Made sales worthy." An executive with a department store chain, Peter joined his mother, Hilda, and his father on weekends, sorting, filling orders, assembling merchandise. "It was decided that to put all our eggs in one basket was a bit too risky, so I didn't join my father immediately. I'd got a family, three little girls."

Hilda, who'd worked in the aircraft industry during World War II, handled the bookkeeping, fully engaged in the new enterprise after years of being "a dutiful

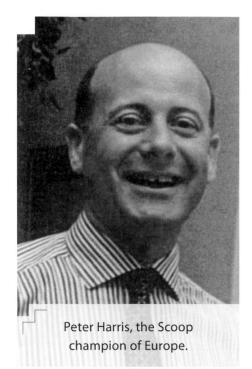

Peter Harris, the Scoop
champion of Europe.

wife in the old-fashioned way, doing what my father wanted." Their quiet married life began many years earlier with a bang and a screech.

Before Appleyard, Leslie Harris had designed planes for the Royal Air Force and during the war "my mum and dad were married in Manchester, which was heavily bombed and almost obliterated." As the newly married couple left the church to go across to the reception, air raid sirens squalled and "they just upped and ran. Bombs were falling but they got across to where they wanted to be." When the dust settled, the reception commenced as planned.

Les and Hilda Harris, according to their son, found a "new lease on life" as they began building the new business together, "supporting each other during the worrying times, as there so often are at the start of a new business." They succeeded faster than they'd expected, and Peter resigned his merchandising job in less than a year to join his parents, traveling around the UK, selling.

And now, it seemed, the intrepid couple had once more got across and were where they wanted to be.

FW Equipment, Ltd. was established in Bradford, England, in 1971. Ferno held 25 percent of the company and Les and his family owned the rest. The new company would sell only Ferno products. That toehold led to an enormous European footprint for Ferno. In 1968, Ferno-Washington's export market represented less than 5 percent of total sales. Four years later, the company gained 80 percent of the UK emergency patient handling equipment market. Then, from 1972 to 1975, the company almost doubled its export volume.

It wasn't simple. The largesse of England's National Health Service led to a brisk use of ambulances, but free transport lowered the threshold for what might be considered an emergency. "Sometimes they'd load three or four people, plus somebody else on a stretcher for one ambulance trip to the hospital. Sometimes it was more like a bus," El said. "We redesigned our cots to fit over the wheel hump and figured out ways to give them more space inside."

Products produced in Wilmington didn't always conform to UK requirements, and Peter tended to tinker with the equipment more than was absolutely necessary, in El's opinion. "Fortunately for us," Peter said, "a group called the Ambulance Service Advisory Committee Setup came up with the ideal stretcher for the UK. A simple design, which wasn't manufactured exactly to those specifications by anybody in the UK or, indeed, anywhere else."

Ferno had a chance to be first into the market with this new product. And they seized that opportunity.

"The Americans produced a prototype called the York One. From that came the York Two, and we sold a few of those. But then Elroy suggested that we include an elevating stretcher trolley, which proved to be the key to success in the UK market. It provided ambulance attendants with the facility to hold to the height of the trolley and reduce the lifting. I remember my first big order. It was some sixty or eighty units. That was a lot in those days. That was the breakthrough. Nobody else in the world had anything like it." The massively popular York Four All Level Cot Bench blended the York One with the Model 30, the elevating X-frame cot.

Jane Fox's ironing board had made its way across the Atlantic.

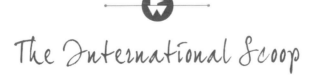

The International Scoop

If the York became England's emergency service workhorse, the Scoop was the racehorse. From the beginning, there was just something wonderfully straightforward about the Scoop. El called it a Wow Product, the value and purpose immediately recognizable. Marvelously simple. Easily managed. Reliably effective. And it could certainly go the distance.

Today, more than forty years after the Scoop made its first UK appearance, rugby teams there have been told by their medical advisers to keep them near the field. "We are advising that players suspected of suffering a spinal injury should be removed from the field with a scoop stretcher rather than the traditional rigid long board," read the advisory. "A scoop stretcher can be split vertically into two parts, with shaped 'blades' toward the center which can be brought together underneath a patient, reducing the chance of undesirable movement of injured areas."

In the hands of Peter Harris, the scoop led the way across Europe during the 1970s. "Peter, without a doubt," El said, "is the world champion in selling our original scoop stretcher concept. He could pick up an injured person on the road, in the grass, laying up against the edge of a wall, and use the scoop just like a surgeon using a tool."

Peter managed, he said, to sell quite a lot of those around the UK, adding that the scoop often "paid for the petrol" when he was pitching other products. "I covered the whole of the UK for a year or two, and then we decided we needed help." Two salesmen were hired, one in the north, one in the south of the UK. Meanwhile, Ferno products were getting attention at UK ambulance exhibits from foreign visitors. Peter started crossing borders.

If you want to take on the job of pioneering Europe, El told him, we'll back you. Ferno will finance you. "He kinda leap frogged around Europe and started to sort out the people that were potential Ferno distributors for us from our customer base," El explained.

"We had the idea of having a warehouse somewhere like Belgium, in Antwerp, because the containers could come in there easily, Peter said. "We created a name called Ferno Europa, but it never really took off." As Peter started rolling through Europe, it became clear to El that local distribution was their best route, that each country had its own regulations, protocols and conditions.

Their early research was fundamental and hands-on. "I got samples from America, loaded them into a big Mercedes diesel van in Holland and toured through Europe to see what the reaction was to these products. I had done some research, but lots of it was seat-of-the-pants stuff, not very sophisticated." Peter settled himself behind the wheel of the truck and spent the next several months singing Beatles songs on the road and jumping through diplomatic hoops at every border.

The European Union was in the distant future. "Every time I went through one border control, I'd have to unload all the stuff, and they'd count it. Then I'd load it, get to the other side, and I'd have to unload it again. They'd count it, check it, and put it back in. It always confused them because the vehicle was German. The stuff was registered in Holland. It was manufactured in America, and I was English."

Once Peter was trying to get out of Belgium into France, where he'd set up an important first meeting with several ambulance company executives. "I got to the border in the evening, and the person on the Belgium side wouldn't let me through, said he hadn't the authority." The "authority" had left for the day. No mobile phones. No computers. No real interest in locating Mr. Big.

"So, I had to leave the van there, get the suitcase out of the front and wheel it all along on the hard shoulder of the motorway until I found a motel. Then wheel it all the way back the next morning to Customs. The right chap was there and boom, boom, boom, I was off." This time.

He began to narrow down his prospects. "The first country to really break through was Holland. Then there was another chap in Belgium, who had some ideas. But it became obvious that the standard USA and UK products wouldn't tick all the boxes for them. We realized that specialization was the way forward."

R&D was the answer, and El set about leading the charge to customize products. Much of the work being done was applicable to other countries, such as Australia and Sweden. Japan would equal the UK as a driving force but in an entirely different way. "They started with the stretcher we developed for Holland, and in their quiet, patient and polite way nudged us to modify and improve it to serve their market," El said.

The notion of Ferno Europa disappeared as El moved toward investing in distribution companies. And in people.

He linked up with entrepreneurs just starting out, finding them in countries where there was no dominant patient handling equipment company. He handpicked the people rather than companies, because the companies didn't exist.

Back in England, Les Harris was making noises about retirement and approached his son about taking over FW Equipment in West Yorkshire, an historic but chilly and land-locked section of England. Peter had moved his family to Antibe, a French resort on the Mediterranean with bragging rights to forty-eight beaches and balmy weather. He told his father he wanted to finish opening up the market in southern Europe. His youngest daughter was just starting school, El was "allowing me to do my own thing, supporting me enormously through research and development. It suited me down to the ground, to be honest."

Les appointed his daughter, Janet Harris. "My sister hadn't had any previous experience in the company, but I think he wanted to keep it in the family. She tried to do the job, telephoned me on a regular basis but it didn't work out." She was gone after a year. El, still a 25 percent shareholder, made a deal with Les in 1980 to buy the rest of the company. Before Les walked out the door for the last time, according to Peter, his father "gave each and every member of staff a huge personal financial award because he felt that he owed the success of the company largely to their efforts."

Peter became managing director and built "a proper big factory." The company was renamed Ferno UK but maintained the same culture. "A very strong family business with good relations with staff and really a pleasure to work at. We continued the idea that we would invest in people who were good family people we would want to be with."

The man who followed Peter as managing director of Ferno UK in 1993, John Wilby, first became aware of Ferno-Washington thirty years earlier when he was an ambulance man in the south of England. Marty McMahon, a Baltimore City firefighter in America, wrote to his British friend about a piece of equipment he considered indispensable. Marty, who became a chief with the department, pulled some strings and sent John a sample in a diplomatic bag.

Wilby went through channels and collected his prize—a Ferno Scoop stretcher.

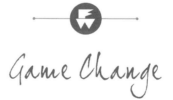

Game Change

While Peter Harris roved Europe in a Mercedes truck, singing Beatles songs at the top of his lungs and looking for ways to sell Ferno products to all of Europe, El was putting together a network of "family people," entrepreneurs to sell and distribute Ferno products around the world. He was financing and organizing new companies and circulating new products aided—and sometimes thwarted— by an industry in the throes of change at home and abroad.

A U.S. report in 1966 created a stir, pointing out that vehicle accidents killed more Americans than were lost in the Korean War and claiming that "if seriously wounded, chances of survival would be better in a combat zone than on the average city street." The combination of poor automobile design and highways lacking proper lighting and signage, along with first responders who were inadequately trained contributed to what President Lyndon Johnson declared "the neglected disease of modern society" as he signed the National Highway Traffic Safety Act, standardizing EMS training.

The white paper, released by the National Academy of Sciences, charged that "adequate ambulance services are as much a municipal responsibility as firefighting and police services." Tending to the sick and wounded was being taken from the hands of funeral directors—a loss most of them welcomed. Maintaining a twenty-four-hour, seven-days-a-week answering service and revving up the hearse in the middle of the night to ride to the site of an auto accident was a service morticians had inherited, particularly in rural areas as physicians stopped making house calls. It was often a thankless job, not to mention costly.

Some funeral directors already had announced that they would no longer make emergency calls. Scott Reinbolt, in his book, *Humble Heroes*, describes an ambulance call from an ailing woman, who insisted that the attendants from the funeral home stop at a laundromat and wait while she washed and dried a fresh outfit to wear to the hospital.

Reeling from a terrible and much publicized train wreck known as the Harrow and Wealdstone Rail Crash, Great Britain had begun restructuring ambulances to become mobile hospitals, rather than simply vehicles to transport patients. Ambulance services were transferred from local authority to central government control in 1974, under regional health authorities. This led to the formation of county based ambulance services. And politics.

El believed combat veterans contributed mightily to the industry around the world. Soldiers came home to find work as firefighters, police officers and ambulance attendants, bringing battlefield trauma lessons to civilian pre-hospital treatment. "We were benefiting from their experiences and what they had to say about patient care." And, of course, El listened.

The focus of emergency care was expanding to include the concerns of the people with their hands on the stretcher. Tending to the needs of the EMTs and other first responders was shown to improve the outcomes for the sick and injured. This was old news to Ferno, which had been listening to funeral directors and ambulance attendants since the days of Dick Ferneau.

"The idea that we looked after not just the patient but the people who looked after the patients had not really clicked yet in Europe," according to Peter Harris.

"The real key was when we were able to make them see that the patient was helped when you make life better and easier for the actual ambulance personnel. People weren't really given very sophisticated tools through which they could accomplish their aims."

In 1982, the Alexander Kielland oil platform collapsed in Norwegian waters, killing 123 people and leading to new focus on medical and rescue equipment throughout Scandinavia. Regulations changed along with equipment, and El had found a nimble emergency response company, small enough to react quickly, large enough to get the job done. Even better, the company's owner was a highly respected former emergency worker who had been tapped by Norwegian authorities to revamp safety standards. Tore Larsen was very much on the inside of a growing demand for better emergency equipment.

He and his wife, Anne Catherine, were the epitome of the brand of entrepreneurs sought by Ferno. As their daughter, Tove, described her parents: "Slowly they were building the company up, bit by bit and piece by piece." Her mother, who'd been running a bookstore in Oslo, took over the finances. And more. "Administrative everything," Anne Catherine said, "from the stock up to the highest level." Tore was traveling, selling, and she handled the accounting, customer service and the care of their three young children. Like Les and Hilda Harris, like El and Elaine Bourgraf, "Together we were a team," she said.

They worked out of their home, out of their cellar, actually. The company, called ScanRescue, was building ambulances to comply with new Norwegian regulations. The ambulances fit regulations. The old stretchers didn't fit the ambulances anymore. They consulted with doctors about the best way to heed the new rules and accommodate medical and space needs inside the vehicles at the same time. The couple started looking around and met El at an American Ambulance Association (AAA) exhibition in Las Vegas.

They clicked. Tore struggled to express his first impressions: "El is a very loyal and very *trustable* person."

"We had an instant connection," Anne Catherine added. "You feel it at once when you meet people." They visited the Bourgrafs in America, then came back again with their children, staying with the Bourgrafs for a few days. Then El loaned them a station wagon, so they could drive down to Disney World. "I think it's a little bit more special to be in a family-operated company, than a shareholder

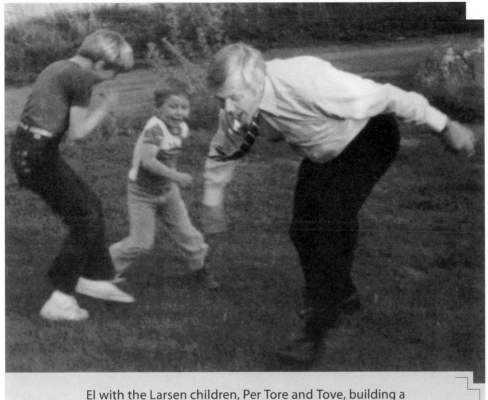

El with the Larsen children, Per Tore and Tove, building a
network of family people.

company. It's much friendlier." Family companies, said Tore, "look at profits in
another way. We have always put the profit back in the company so it grows instead
of using too much money ourselves."

Tore added, "And you have direct contact to the chairman you know."

They had much in common, these two families with their kids and their
work ethic. And they shared an absolute faith in their ability to succeed. Failure
"was never in our mind," Anne Catherine insisted. Ever. "Nobody should enter
a business if they are not wholehearted with it," Tore said. "It's not 8 to 4 o'clock
work. It's twenty-four hours a day."

The Larsens felt ready to tackle the sprawl of the Nordic countries—Sweden,
Denmark, Finland and Iceland, along with their native Norway, a small population
but geographically daunting. They wanted exclusive rights to sell Ferno products
throughout Scandinavia. There was one hitch, and it was serious. Tore was still
building ambulances, as well as selling the equipment for them.

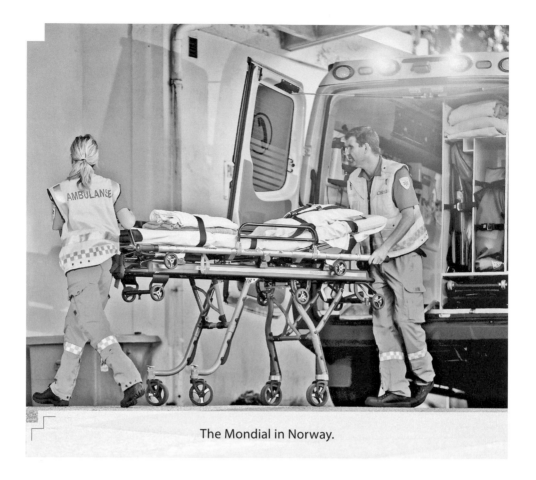

The Mondial in Norway.

"Exclusive was the key word," El said. "We just could not give an ambulance builder total control over the right to sell our products. It just wouldn't work. It had to be with a company that could sell to all ambulance builders, and it's difficult to work both sides of the street, to sell to a competitor."

This might have been a bitter pill to swallow. It was, after all, a major redirection for Tore Larsen. But El and Tore had history. And trust.

In 1979, with support from El, the Larsens founded Ferno Norden, quickly cementing their reputation for quality emergency equipment with exclusive rights to Ferno products. After the Kielland disaster, Ferno Norden was a key supplier of not only stretchers but several types of emergency products, including lights. They also rebuilt cars, retrofitting standard automobiles for use as police cars or emergency vehicles.

The Larsens had a tested ally in place as they expanded their customer base. It started with a Jaws-of-Life type rescue tool belonging to a Swedish salesman named Hans Andersson. Tore watched a demonstration at a Stockholm show and wanted to sell the tool back home in Norway. "He didn't have any money with him," Hans said, "but I took a chance on him." Tore carried off ten, sold ten and came back to pay Hans and buy twenty more tools. Then he returned a week later to buy another fifty. Soon after that, Tore asked Hans if he'd like to add stretchers to his product lineup.

Tore knew of some very good ones, made in America, by the Ferno-Washington Company.

"I had no clue where I could sell the stretchers," Hans chuckled. He went home and pawed through the telephone directory to no avail. But he'd been working with the Volvo company, testing the strength of the sedan's doors with his rescue tool. He called his contact there, saying he was now in the stretcher business.

The voice on the other end of the line went quiet for a second.

"Ambulance stretchers?"

"Yes."

"I want 106 of them," the Volvo man said.

Hans placed a hurried call to Tore. Two hours later they met in Sweden, fixed on a price, a model and a delivery date—three weeks, working night and day, promised Tore, as soon as Volvo signed the contract. The automotive executives were at a retreat, so Hans joined them in the hotel sauna and got a name on a slightly damp dotted line. Back in Wilmington, the Ferno workers went into action—delivering 106 perfectly turned out Ferno stretchers, right on deadline.

"That was the start of Sweden Rescue," Hans said. "So Tore started on a product I was selling, and I started my company by a product he was selling. So there is a connection."

And, as usual, the connection expanded to include the Bourgrafs. All of them. Hans and his wife, Gunilla, and the Larsens were invited to visit the factory where the stretchers were made. "I had never met El before and not Elaine either. So when we came there, they picked us up in a Lincoln Town Car, the biggest, longest car I ever saw in my life," Hans said.

They continued on to Wilmington for a tour. "We met a lot of nice people working there. I think they thought we were a little exotic coming from Norway and Sweden, because they were asking us very strange questions—if it was dark all year, or if it was very far from the North Pole, and if there were bears on the streets."

After that, they drove to the Bourgrafs' home in Cincinnati, where Joe taught Hans how to throw an American football and El talked him into competing in a neighborhood lawn mower race. Gunilla and Hans were escorted downstairs to the faux pickle stand.

"I thought it was so fantastic," Hans said, "to see how this family wanted to remember their roots. It was nice to see, very nice to see. And you build up what I like to call relations. We were a small company. We had just started. And they took care of us in a very special way. They let us into their family. We have the same values they have. So we fit together. We trust each other. El and me, well, we had the feeling we could work together. That feeling we still have."

From those first stretchers, Hans built an ambulance business that sold units all over the world—from Jamaica to Yugoslavia, from Kuwait to the Philippines. He has since sold Sweden Rescue and his eleven other rescue-based companies and now invests in start-up companies. "We have been living on the first order of those stretchers for forty years. The foundation of all of this, of our life is Ferno."

Ferno was putting its stamp on quality companies all over the globe, with the inveterate Bourgraf spin and focus. FW Equipment Australia, the only company in that country to specialize in emergency and safety products, took the name Ferno Australia in 1974 when it became a fully owned subsidiary. The company still is managed by descendants of its founder, the late Ken Ferris.

Ken's wife, Carol, also worked by his side, along with his daughter Lucia Brankovich. His son, Alan, and his nephew, Scott West, who are Ferno Australia former and current directors, join an astonishing number of successful Ferno subsidiaries which have family at their core.

Local distributors were used in smaller countries, such as Spain, Portugal, Holland and Belgium, but in the larger markets, Ferno established a distinct presence, and, although each bore the parent company's name, each firm's title paid deference to the country of origin. Eventually, there would be a Ferno Canada, Ferno France, Ferno Italy, Ferno Japan, Ferno Slovakia, and Ferno Transportgeräte in Germany.

"We invested our money in these companies to give them the assurance of continuity of supply," Peter Harris said, "and the assurance that we weren't just looking for a quick fix, to sell something today, and then leave them in the lurch tomorrow."

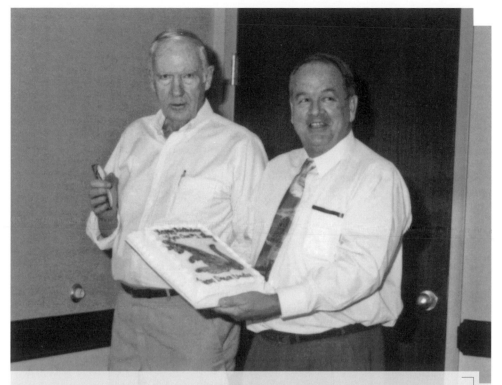

Dick and Ken Ferris, first Managing Director of Ferno Australia, 1974–1997.

Olaf Matnusson said his small company, Donna, in Iceland, relied on Ferno Norden and the Larsens not only to sell him quality products, but to provide him with quality information. "We are only 300,000 people living in Iceland with seventy ambulances." Olaf could not afford any buying mistakes. Tore kept him abreast of regulatory changes in the wind and made sure that his Ferno purchases would withstand both the harsh Icelandic winters and the sometimes equally harsh regulatory scrutiny. And, not incidentally, improve the lives of the users.

Tore, who worked on a Red Cross rescue team before he began selling equipment, was a kindred soul. El praised Tore's "tenacity in pursuit of the customer" and his skill in juggling the needs and contacts in five distinct countries. "It isn't just getting the first order, it's making sure you keep your promises so you'll get the second, third, and fourth."

El was taking the long view—just as he and Dick had done when they made the decision back in Greenfield to sell to wholesale outlets only—expanding the Ferno family, working *with* them.

Frequent Flyer Milestones

Jon Ellis, who collected his first paycheck from Ferno UK when he was 16 years old, recollected the first time he traveled to Wilmington. "I was in the Blue Room—the R&D area—when I saw Elroy for the first time. Dick Ferneau was with him." Working on a new product, both men stopped to shake hands with Jon and exchange pleasantries. The Brit was amazed at the attention from the company's top brass. More amazed to see them working on the shop floor.

"I thought, these two guys get involved at the heart of the business, looking at solutions, pushing with the team, wanting feedback from their employees."

Jon would remain with Ferno for thirty years, becoming one of the company's most influential and successful managing directors. What he saw in the Blue Room was a way of doing business that may have begun in Wilmington but has been translated into a company culture that is exported throughout the world.

"I've traveled," Jon said, "and seen a lot of the Ferno group operations in a lot of places, and I get the same feeling everywhere." The key, he said, is "an open door—an organization caring for its employees." Ferno develops its people, listens to them and encourages them to push the boundaries. The result, he said, is "you won't believe what people do to make the company a success."

Jon cites the flexibility he was given to work with UK customers both in government and in the private sector. "Ferno really wanted to understand their business, provide solutions. Sometimes we would modify a product to meet their specific needs. Or we may push the boat out and create a complete new product for that customer."

"Elroy always wanted somebody who actually was a native of the country to run things," said Gary Hiles, who went from paperboy to gofer to Ferno's Vice President of International Sales during the mid-1980s. "We'd try to incorporate the Ferno U.S. ideas, but then El always tried to adapt it to the way it worked within their country." He respected them, and their culture. And they knew it.

"I definitely feel very much part of the Ferno team," said Scott West of Ferno Australia. "At the same time, we are encouraged to be entrepreneurial."

Helen McFadden, Gary's executive secretary, said when she started working at Ferno in 1985, Ferno had international visitors at least twice a month. El Bourgraf, as usual, set the tone. And the tone was at once welcoming and businesslike. Visitors were greeted by the sight of their own country's flag flying next to the American flag atop the administration building. Helen said she liked to imagine their thoughts when they saw it. "When they came down Airport Road to look up and see their flag, I think that just says welcome in the biggest way."

Visitors were tightly scheduled—another mark of esteem, Helen said. "They'd traveled thousands of miles, over oceans, and we wanted it to be enjoyable—and very productive. When they left, we wanted them to feel like they'd accomplished everything they wanted to achieve while they were here."

Meals and accommodations were arranged, Helen said, "to make them realize that this was their company and their home when they were in the United States—when they were here in Wilmington."

Not all foreign visitors were customers or employees. Some were bureaucrats, government officials, trying to work on improving the emergency services in their countries.

"We actually help establish all the standards from the top level, from the departments of health, the ministries of health," Gary explained. "We provide backup material—how to build an ambulance, what equipment should go inside. We have that knowledge base, and we share that with these developing countries. We do a lot of groundbreaking—all the details upfront to make sure that once they're ready to implement the process and the system, it's ready to go."

When Turkey needed help with its EMS service, a contingent came to Wilmington. Almost all of them were smokers. "We had no smokers here in our company," Gary said. El told them, "I realize you guys smoke, and you're very, very important to us. So, I will allow you to smoke in our cafeteria, but you can't smoke anyplace else."

The Turks chose to take their tobacco outside. "They didn't smoke in our building," Gary said. "Now, if you think about that, that's like Elroy giving them an olive branch. You're important to us. We respect you as our customer. But what was even nicer was, they respected him. That's one thing that Elroy was always able to do. He let people know how he felt and that was that he respected everybody for what they were, and what they could be."

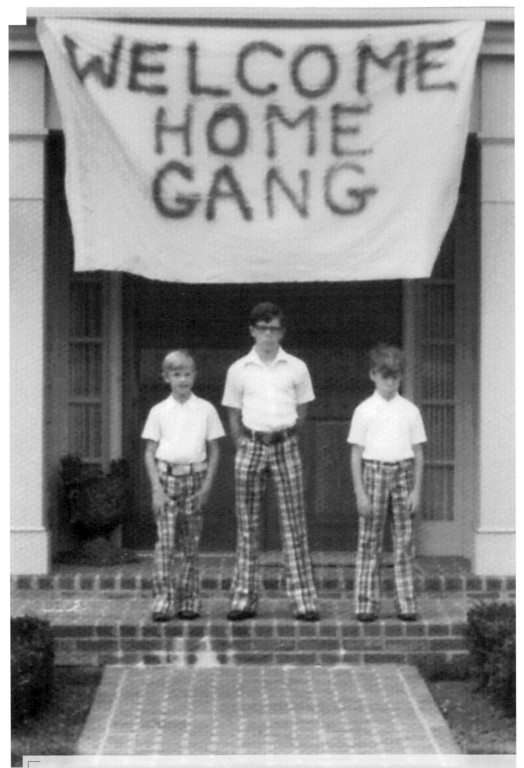

The Bourgraf boys joined their parents in welcoming international visitors.

El was always the essential El. Respectful. Courteous. And unabashedly, perpetually a family man. He was quick to fold newcomers into the family.

"El knew everybody, their wives, their kids, anniversaries, birthdays," Gary said. "It goes back to Elroy's values as a person—his family, his faith, and his community." When he talks about the Ferno family, he says, it extends to about a thousand people worldwide. "El and Elaine always opened their home. So, too, did Gary and his wife, Sharon.

"I still remember what we fed Rolf Steinmetz when he came for dinner," Gary said. Rolf, the very German leader of Ferno's German subsidiary, was treated to a typical American family meal—spaghetti. Not only that, Rolf attended his first Oktoberfest not in Bavaria but in Cincinnati, Ohio.

El had met Rolf earlier, introduced by Peter Harris. Harkening back to his German years in the Army, El said he "knew something about the German intellect, the way they thought, the ones who were productive and the ones who were the followers. I saw that independence in Rolf, that he was not afraid to challenge me on anything, yet he was willing to learn something about our business and how he could apply those principles in Germany."

They started doing business. El said he appreciated Rolf's ability to "listen before he talks. And he understands what he wants to say before he says it. That's Rolf from day one." Rolf, like Tore and Anne Catherine, found El to be very "trustable." Sometimes their contracts were on a handshake. Sometimes, El joked, they were written on a cocktail napkin, damp with stout German beer.

Rolf, who began as an intern in Cologne, Germany, with a company that manufactured first-aid equipment and stretchers, had founded a company called Feruta with his boss to sell Ferno products directly to end users, bypassing dealers. According to Peter Harris, they'd been frustrated by buyers who were not particularly warm to the concerns of the emergency personnel. There were no wheels on German rescue equipment. "We don't roll people along." Peter and Rolf were told. The hard-nosed attitude was, "I pay my people to carry, and they'll carry."

Before he added Ferno products to his line, Rolf said, "We just had a stretcher you had to carry—two poles and four handles." Customers told Rolf that the Ferno products didn't conform to German standards. Which they didn't. Ferno was light years ahead of that standard. And not cheap. So Rolf looked for buyers who had faith in the product and enough clout to ignore the bureaucrats. End users.

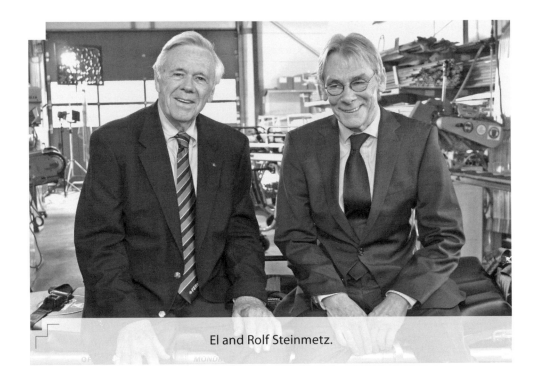

El and Rolf Steinmetz.

A turning point, Rolf said, was getting the Frankfurt Fire Service to switch over to Ferno. "We gave them three stretchers, and they tested them for two months, then asked for another one, which they did not get free of cost."

Frankfurt started with a Model 30. Then came an order for the Roll-In System (the Multi-Level Model 35) after the fire chief saw it at a convention. Two years later, the service equipped its entire fleet of ambulances with Ferno equipment. A big win. A milestone. Then came big ambulance services in Munich and Hanover. After ten years, Rolf even managed to win over the uber-strict Deutsches Institut fur Normung (DIN), the German Institute for Standardization.

"When we started demonstrating the Ferno roll-in stretchers, we got the same comments from our customers again and again: 'This stretcher is not to DIN.' One day when Peter and I were on a demo tour, Peter made a small drawing showing a DINosaur and underlined the DIN.

"From that day on, we viewed the members of the DIN board as dinosaurs—old fashioned, slowly disappearing creatures. One day we put it in an advertisement: 'The time of the DINosaur is gone. The wheel has been invented, but the stretchers are still the same.' Then the unbelievable happened—the DIN board started making their own specifications for a wheeled stretcher. We managed to bring the DINosaurs to today's standards. We put wheels under the German stretcher regulations without even being a member of the DIN board."

"Rolf is very patient," El laughed.

Feruta became Ferno's German subsidiary, Ferno Transportgerate, maintaining the original business model. "We offer the customer a free demonstration and let him test the product. After sales, we offer him free instructions, show him how to work this product, and we have a service center so if there is a problem, we can react very fast and solve it."

By now, Ferno was a juggernaut in Europe, with a new subsidiary and a host of products developed for this new market. Gary Hiles was ready in the wings to take the company to the next level.

"I traveled domestically for Elroy until '83, when he decided he didn't want to travel internationally as much, so I said hey, why not? And he's a good teacher," Gary said. "So he just transformed me from a domestic guy to an international guy."

Gary already knew some of the international customers, thanks to El's transworld shuttle. "There was already a lot of interaction between international and domestic customers. I just followed El's lead, listened to what he said about other cultures." Some of it was simple. "He taught me the proper way to bow to the Japanese. He reminded me never to take our Jewish customers to a rib joint." But that was the small stuff. He told his protégé to "keep your eye on the target, keep your priorities straight, and concentrate on major issues. The details will take care of themselves."

Elroy was still leading Gary up the mountain. And pointing out the scenery.

He had an extremely apt pupil. Back when Gary was working at his "interim" job at Ferno, taking inventory and waiting to get a real job offer, El sent the young man to Dr. Lucien Cohen, Burt Weil's old friend and a renowned industrial psychologist. Go see him, El told Gary. "If he says you're OK, I'll give you a shot. If not, you'll have a direction in life." Cohen administered a thorough battery of tests measuring intelligence, values, interests, knowledge, personality traits, and skills. Not only did Gary measure up, but El's investment of time and money was an indication of the future he envisioned for his former paperboy.

The domestic to international sales education began long before Gary stepped into the job.

"Elroy never made you guess. You always had all the information he did." And that was a lot of information. "Elroy traveled all the time, listened to everybody. He picked up a lot of new, creative, different ideas every time he sat next to somebody on a plane. He got outside exposure to other companies, to make us better. When he'd go on a trip, we would be back at the shop wondering what the next big idea would be."

And they were ready to climb on board, excited to follow his lead. "When Elroy walked into the room, everybody in the industry knew who he was and respected him. Ferno set the standards. There's no other company in the industry that actually has new and different products. They all copy Ferno." Dating back, he said, to the early days. "Elroy and Dick Ferneau are the guys that have driven this industry from day one—initially from the mortuary, now to the global EMS business. It's all around Elroy's vision and work and the good people he has been able to attract," Gary said.

If there are a thousand ways to do something, he continued, El will find a thousand and one. "If you look globally at our industry, there's not one innovative thought that wasn't generated by Ferno, not one that doesn't come from here. Elroy never copied anything—he just improved it. Ferno is a brand that reflects the man. He never lets us forget that we might transport your mother or father or your child. We want to make sure the product we supply is the best; that it functions as it's supposed to."

"I don't know of any other company in the world that can say they started an industry, developed that industry and as long as we've been around, we have been the leader of that industry. You are your own competitor. You have to come up with the new ideas."

When Gary casts an eye toward expanding the business globally, he said he simply watches for an improving quality of life. "As countries evolve toward better health care for their citizens, we know they will need our products." Developing countries use many of Ferno's original designs. "They don't have the infrastructure or trained personnel to use some of our latest designs. But we'll be ready when they do. They usually come to us. Our brand is known. We provide equipment free of charge to schools, and we work with them to satisfy their needs." Which can vary greatly.

"We have the knowledge base, and then we share that with these developing countries. We are involved in all the specification writing for Europe and Asia. We've just implemented the European standard now in India."

He ticked off international progress on the fingers of both hands. Israel is 100 percent Ferno products. So is Jordan, England, Ireland and Norway. "You go to South Africa, you go to Australia, you go to Japan…You go to any country in Europe. Eastern Europe, Ferno has an influence. South America—Ferno has influence. He has his sights set on the BRIC countries—Brazil, Russia, India, and China.

"So many opportunities," he said with relish.

And just like his mentor, he was ready to hit the gas. Forward. Drive.

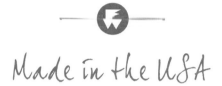

Made in the USA

Ferno comfortably straddled several continents by the mid-1980s. With Gary Hiles turning up the heat on international emergency and rescue sales, El went into a brand new mode—building and diversifying, exploring new domestic territory.

It seemed to El a natural progression. An attitude. A vision. "Otherwise, we'd just be two small companies in two small towns," he said. The hundreds of trade shows, the thousands of customer calls, listening, translating customer questions into new products and improvements on old ones. It was commercial treasure, not to be squandered. "Aggressive yet personal service has been responsible for increasing our sales volume every year since the company began in 1955."

Energized and confident, bolstered by "the sales effort that placed our products in front of buyers and users throughout the world," he was ready for new markets and new products.

In January of 1983, Ferno signed a deal with Beatrice Foods to buy two of its health care properties, the Market Forge Health Company in Wilmington, Massachusetts, and Forge's Ille Division in Williamsport, Pennsylvania. Ferno had been manufacturing supply carts for in-hospital use for the Market Forge label for several years. El was intrigued by the company's history and its possibilities.

Market Forge started out in Boston, hammering and twisting metal into meat hooks in the 1800s. Over time, a new generation of products emerged from the workshop of founder and blacksmith Louis Beckwith. He was hired to build galvanized racks to replace unsanitary food storage on wooden shelves in restaurants and institutions. In the late 1920s, the company began using stainless steel and produced the first modern steam cooker, leading to other products for the food, nursing home and hospital industries.

When the health service division caught El's eye, it was producing medication preparation and transport systems, sterilizing equipment, mortuary tables, and surgical scrub stations.

Beatrice's Ille Division had a colorful beginning and a similarly circuitous route to health care. During the 1920s, the company was known for its exercise equipment. Founder F. Wilson Ille hired Charles Atlas, the circus strongman famous for comic book ads depicting him as a 97-pound weakling bullied at the beach before he buffed up with exercise. Atlas demonstrated a spring-pull device supposedly responsible for his bulging biceps in the window of Ille's Manhattan store. From there, Ille partnered with a physician to develop whirlpool hydrotherapy treatments in stainless steel tanks, leading to a product line of paraffin baths, burn tubs, Sitz baths, and electric bed tents.

In 1985, Ferno built a 70,000-square-foot addition to the 40,000-square-foot Ferno Ille plant in Pennsylvania, closing the Massachusetts plant and transplanting Ferno Forge to the Allegheny Mountains. "We broke ground in April, moved in in September," remembered the no-nonsense Dave Haines. "Most people would've spent two years planning the architectural drawings. We built it in a few months, and there was a crack in the floor but it was okay."

Moving Forge was a Hail Mary attempt to fix it. El called the acquisition "one of my biggest mistakes. I didn't do my due diligence, and we paid for it." One problem was the receivables. Forge estimators had worked with architects for new facilities that were two or three years away from completion. Hospitals and clinics, for instance, would be designed with wall recesses for work stations, with plumbing and electric infrastructure ready to receive finished stainless steel cabinets and tables.

Trouble was "there were no escalator clauses in the contracts," El said ruefully, "and by the time they were ready for the stations to be installed, costs had gone up." Ferno honored quotes in the original contracts, and lost money or, at best, broke even on every one.

The Market Forge division was producing more headaches than profits, including key suppliers. The steelworkers of Boston were unmoved by El's charm. "I thought I could Ferno-ize them." He'd started making weekly visits to the plant, the last one was when a huge sheet of steel dropped right behind him. "This seemed like a good time to get out of town," he said.

Three years later, Ferno announced the relocation of Ferno Ille to Ohio and sold Forge to MDT, Inc. Like an interesting cousin just slightly out of step with the rest of the family, Forge never transitioned beyond its original ice and nourishment stations, operating room cabinets and surgical scrub sinks. El and Bernie had gotten costs under control but "the product lines do not fit in with the company's future plans. Every employee is being offered further employment options," said a Ferno memo.

There would be plenty of space for the Ille machinery and workers at the Wilmington headquarters, which had grown as needed since opening in 1972. From the original 80,000 square feet, an engineering building had been added in 1974. That same year, warehouse space, four metal buildings and a parking lot were added. More space was added to shipping in 1985. Sometimes, like the Williamsport project, it was done in a hurry. And maybe more practical than pretty.

This time, El was re-imagining and re-designing the abandoned Air Force building into an international headquarters. This time there were architectural drawings.

First, of course, he listened to his Ferno family. Helen McFadden, Gary Hiles' long-time secretary, was fairly new to the company and remembers her delight at filling out a questionnaire sent out to employees asking what they'd like to have in the new building. "Everybody wanted a window because we didn't have them in the old building."

El was also keenly aware of what the company needed to stay competitive, and this building reflected his scrupulous business practices. He ordered an exhaustive review and usage forecast by Ferno's special projects manager, Bill Wilson. "The past five-year history indicates 100 new or modified products per year from, say, a simple latch to a totally new concept," Wilson said in his report. He allowed a certain number of manufacturing square feet per product, then multiplied out the years and costs and came up with a recommendation.

Peter Harris may have gauged the European market "by the seat of his pants," but El never did.

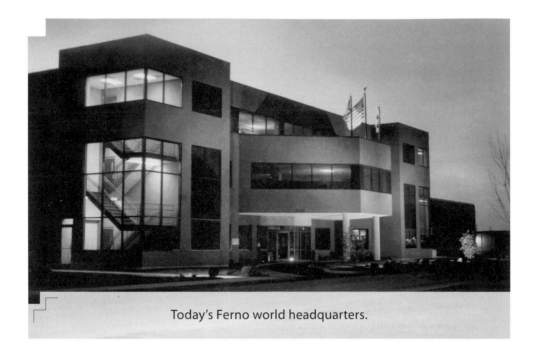

Today's Ferno world headquarters.

"He never went off the deep end," was the way Gary Hiles described his mentor. "He thought things through." El paired facts and figures and logic with his instincts. And he got his money's worth from his degree at the University of Cincinnati's School of Business.

George Reazer, who was vice president of manufacturing, said, "We were aware of competition. We had high work standards, and we were very interested in the quality of the products we shipped. We were also interested in shipping products on time." One priority for this new building was adding more space for shipping and manufacturing.

In 1987, El hired Cincinnati architect George Paul, whose previous work included Garfield Tower and the Vernon Manor Hotel, and who was a Beta Theta Pi brother at the University of Cincinnati. It was to be his last project. Paul died two years later at the age of 62. In his obituary, his widow told of Paul's favorite work—designing a home for a paraplegic "that made her self-sufficient for the first time in her life." His son, Mark, who took over the business, said his father's philosophy was always that an architectural product should be a true partnership between a client and an architect."

It was no mystery as to why El Bourgraf might have chosen this particular designer. And there may have been the typical collegial Bourgraf partnership, but El knew exactly what he wanted and needed with this project, which would result in more than a quarter of a million square feet of space under one roof. This was a big move, and he was determined to do it without losing sales or missing deadlines.

He had sketched it out in several precise phases, first enlarging shipping and manufacturing, then connecting the existing three buildings. Then he'd wave the Ille operation through the doors and, finally, erect a three-story brick and glass administrative complex. The new headquarters would include a conference room, training facility with audio-visual capabilities, and a cafeteria. There would be an interior courtyard with a fountain.

And windows. Plenty of windows.

Bob Ginter kept a faithful scrapbook of the nuts and bolts building process, including stacks of bricks on wood pallets and a graphic account of the new HVAC system being lowered onto the roof by crane—"Whew! Made it!" He also collected a few sentimental photographs—one closeup of a hyacinth with twisted rebar and construction rubble in the background and another picture that he noted was "the last piece of grass." Not to worry. By the time he finished, El would have new grass, landscaping and a newly paved parking lot.

After the Ille division was relocated, the administrative offices came to life, designed with glass on both the front and back. Vacated offices became homes to support groups, such as engineering and research and development. Temperature-controlled environments were built to satisfy the requirements of computer systems and a computer-assisted design center was installed.

By the summer of 1989, Ferno's new international headquarters was ready for company, beginning in August with a reception for state and local officials, a cookout for employees and their families, and another reception for vendors, customers, dealers, and distributors. It was friendly, familial and international all at the same time, with crew that started in Washington Court House, as well as representatives from Japan, Australia, England, West Germany, Turkey, Norway, Mexico, Belgium and Nigeria.

The tail end of Bob's careful record: "Inside Ferno-Washington, you will find a proud workforce that is concerned with quality and committed to excellence. Here is where raw materials become tools for patient rescue, where men and women dedicate their lives' work to lifesaving equipment."

The Family Tree

From a March, 1983, *Ferno Scoop...* "published for and by the employees of Ferno-Washington, Inc.":

This special edition has been put together for the purpose of introducing each of our four divisions to each other and to welcome the new members of the Ferno Family. Why do we say the Ferno Family, instead of "the employees"? Well, for one thing, we like to include the entire family of our people in the process of our communication. For this reason, there is frequently family contact, and the Scoop *is sent to home addresses, so that other family members can enjoy what is happening at work. In addition to this, we believe that the people who work at Ferno and the people who run it actually think like a family.*

Sound cornball? Think for a moment about some families you know and what makes their relationships different from relationships between non-family members. For one, they think as a team. Not that they don't ever disagree, but that they considered each other before acting and tried to work toward a common purpose (such as providing long-term career employment or producing a quality product). In addition to simply thinking like a team, families care about each other. Having "grown up" together in a supportive environment, the relationship is more than just economic and gets into mutual trust and respect. We really want this feeling to drift naturally from Ferno-Washington into the new divisions, from the personnel practices to the way in which every day operating decisions are made.

The key to making this happen is communication—up, down, and across. Those who call the shots need to know what their people are thinking, and those who have to live by the decisions need to know why that particular course of action is necessary. While a monthly newsletter helps somewhat, this communication would really take place every day—on the plant floor or in the office—whether by conversation, suggestions, meetings, bulletins, or whatever. It takes all the folks at Ferno to make this happen.

The essay was unsigned. No by-line was necessary. It was pure Elroy Bourgraf.

"You keep hearing about the Ferno family, part of the big culture here," said Paul Riordan, the company's chief financial officer. "It's really a true belief that it is a family-type deal. You see that in the way the Bourgrafs treat us and the way people work together. You can have disagreements but at the end of the day you make a decision and you just move on. Lots of places, that doesn't happen. It's just a good working environment full of friendly people with honest integrity. I've been here eighteen years, so I know what I'm talking about."

He got a sense of the way things were going to shape up during his first month on the job, learning that customers also were folded into the Ferno family. "We had a customer who owed us a sizable amount of money. They'd been a distributor of ours for more than twenty

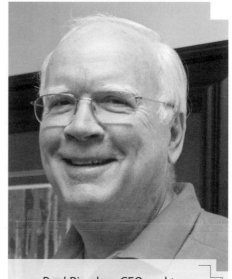

Paul Riordan, CFO and true believer in the "family-type deal."

years. El asked me to work out a deal with them so that we could get our money but it wouldn't hurt them."

Suppliers, too, were treated with respect. "If we were having tight cash flow or anything like that, we had to take care of them. Employees see how customers, suppliers—everybody—is treated like part of this organization. We're here to succeed and be loyal to each other, and if something goes wrong, you jump in, you help them out, and you don't leave people stranded out there. If we have a product that's a problem, we take care of it right away. We don't mess around. We wouldn't do like some of the big car companies do—leave these problems out there until people are injured."

George Reazer, hired as director of engineering before he was put in charge of manufacturing, describes the main attitude as a "composite of the personalities of the employees." Beginning with El. Open. Inclusive.

"The company employees would let outsiders in. When I came and hadn't gone to their school system, hadn't lived in southern Ohio for the first part of my life, I was well received."

But what about the really *inside* insiders, the ones who grew up in the Bourgraf home? Joe, Brian, and El-B? "The boys never took the position, 'well, my dad owns the company, and I can do whatever I want to do,'" George said. "In fact, it was probably more the reverse—that Dad owned the company, and we'd better do what Dad thinks is right to support Ferno."

Dad had definite ideas about the way it would work.

First, there was the grinding room. It was not a metaphor. It was real. It was noisy. It was dirty. And it was where all three Bourgraf sons started their Ferno careers. El-B, the youngest son, spent a year there, smoothing out rough edges left during the metal fabrication—the casting—process. Parts cast elsewhere were shipped to the Ferno plant for finishing. "You'd go home at night literally black," he said. "Dirt was on our faces. Clothes just filthy. You couldn't touch anything."

Joe, the oldest son, who now runs the company, said none of the three sons was pushed toward a Ferno career. The push all three remember most was toward education. After Summit, Joe attended Indian Hill High School then finished high school at Culver Military Academy in Indiana, something he called "an exceptional opportunity." The school, which has nurtured CEOs, as well as entertainers such as country singer Dierks Bentley and actor Hal Holbrook, not to mention sports figures George Steinbrenner and Roger Penske, has a 99 percent college matriculation rate.

"It allowed me to grow personally and also provided an enormous amount of structure and taught me certain characteristics that I continue today." Polished shoes. A certain bearing that, while it might not strike observers as military, it certainly has a robust air of command and leadership. After graduation from Culver in 1979, Joe studied at Miami University, then earned a bachelor's degree in marketing from Xavier University.

He began selling computers and software for a Cincinnati company, then was recruited by Sperry Corporation, which merged with Burroughs Corporation to form Unisys Corporation. Joe climbed the corporate ladder to become the senior exec for the flight management software redesign for Continental and Eastern Airlines.

"It all interwove from the early days of the personal computer to large systems at large corporations, with technology that controlled grand systems—airlines, banks, governmental operations."

El-B said he became more comfortable in the shop than in the administrative offices. "I'm more like Uncle Dick," he said. A St. Xavier High School graduate, he "bounced around college" for a while—Spring Hill College in Alabama, and closer to home, Wilmington College, the University of Cincinnati and Xavier University.

Then he started his own painting business with a friend. For the next four and a half years, he worked on houses and commercial buildings, then came back to Ferno. To the grinding room. He moved to cots assembly, then became a supervisor for the next fifteen years or so, in both cots and the sheet metal department. A year-long stint in Europe, then back to Wilmington to work in engineering and R&D. Then he took over the mortuary division marketing. "Besides my dad, I think I am the Bourgraf who has worked the longest at the company."

El said of his youngest son, "El-B earned his own stripes. He stands high, in my opinion. He didn't have the accounting business background, but acquired some of that by association. And he inherited some of the Kunkel-Bourgraf people skills. "He did not have one enemy in the plant. Employees still hold him in high regard."

The company was making money, and Brian was the "lucky guy who got to give some of it away," working through the Ferno and the Bourgraf Family Foundation to "help out" in Clinton, Highland and Fayette counties, where most of Ferno's American employees live. Often the face of Ferno-Washington, Brian has not only dispensed money but has served on boards including Habitat for Humanity, Little Hearts Big Smiles, Community Care Hospice and the Red Cross. After graduation from Purcell Marian High School in Cincinnati, he came to Wilmington College to collect his undergraduate degree.

After school, he took a job with a tool manufacturer, the Irwin Auger Bit Company in Wilmington, working in human resources and community relations, then in marketing and accounting before landing back at Ferno. Irwin, which has since been absorbed by Rubbermaid and moved to North Carolina, gave Brian the chance to find his own niche.

His health, understandably, has dramatically shaped his life. But, he would argue, not diminished it. "I skied. I swam. I played soccer and traveled." The "kidney thing," as he puts it, has made him a better friend, a better husband and father, a more empathetic human being. "I'm just a lucky guy."

The "lucky guy," of course, also did his time in the grinding room.

Listed in the Guinness Book of World Records as the longest surviving double kidney transplant patient, Brian's luck seemed to run out in 2011. After forty-three years, "I was at work and I just felt something go, and I ran to El-B's office." His brother rushed him to the hospital, and he was put on dialysis, which continued for seven months while he waited for a new kidney.

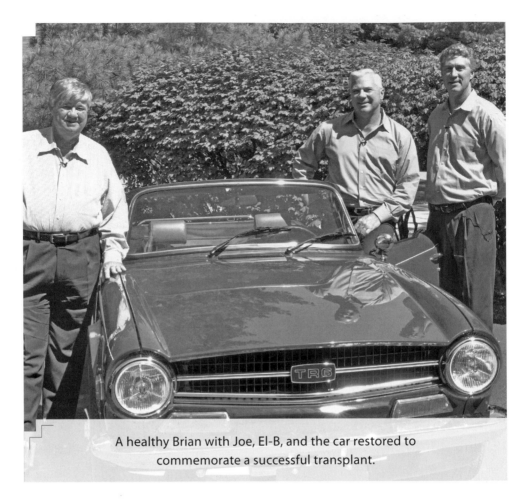

A healthy Brian with Joe, El-B, and the car restored to commemorate a successful transplant.

Potential donors were lining up. People from the plant. People from the community. People from his family, including Joe's son, Zach. "I'll never forget that," Brian said, "I asked if he'd talked to his parents."

"Ahhh, don't worry about that," his nephew said. "I read about it on the Internet. Let's get on with it. What's a few days of pain for me, versus you on a machine?" Both he and his brother, Chris, matched. So did a woman who worked in the plant. But it was Joe Bourgraf who, as he put it "had the honor."

Traveling in Asia, when he received word of Brian's crisis, the eldest Bourgraf son was tested immediately. "We're very blessed that we could facilitate both the physical donation as well as the financial and mental preparation for it. Quite honestly, he probably saved my life. I was hard charging, high cholesterol, high liver enzymes and high blood pressure." He did for his brother what he had not been doing for himself. He exercised, lost weight, got fit.

While Joe was in the hospital for the surgery, El-B stole his car. It was a 1976 Triumph TR6, a British six-cylinder sports car. Joe had been meaning to restore it for more than twenty years.

"My wife said, 'you know what, Joe is doing a really nice thing for Brian. Let's do something really nice for him.'" El-B and his wife, Mary, found a place in Cincinnati that would help them with a restoration. They stripped the car down "to its bare bones and re-plated, repainted, redid it—a 100 percent restoration," El-B said.

Not a possible donor, it was what he could do.

"I'll never forget the day Joe and Brian were in for surgery for Brian's kidney transplant. You could have heard a pin drop in any hallway of this company," said Dorothy Deaton, Ferno's vice president of legal and regulatory compliance. "We were all waiting for that phone call saying they were both fine."

Brian's first day back at work, he walked through the plant. Somebody started to clap. Then people stood up. Brian looked around and saw faces he'd known since childhood. The applause continued. It got louder.

It was a family thing.

"This company is just a good corporate neighbor…They've probably helped every charity in town at one time or another… Ferno has stood by the people of this community. With jobs. With good jobs."

5

Corporate Character

Inside Jokes

Ish and Henry. The fond and familiar nicknames of Ferno's founders are part of company lore. One of El's Army buddies, "a guy named Ernie from Georgia who came from a wealthy family" used to drag El on weekend shopping trips when he was stationed in Germany. They'd enter a place that sold, say, fantastic china or costly antiques. Both were in uniform, and to serve notice to the shop owner that they were serious customers, Ernie would point to El and announce dramatically, *Ish habse feilgelt*, German for, "He has much money."

The phonetic mash-up was abbreviated and Americanized. Ish. The nickname stuck and, thanks to Bernie Zoldak, made its way to America. Dick Ferneau, tickled with the story and the sound, used it in personal correspondence with El. In turn, El called his partner "Henry." Dick's full name was Richard H. Ferneau. "He'd never say what his middle initial stood for, so I just fixed on the name Henry," El said. "It was just between us. Personal. Nobody else called him that." And like M.Z. Klever, Dick took the secret of the name on his birth certificate to his grave.

Most institutions, if they have any personality at all, are replete with nicknames and inside jokes, incidents told over and over again, amid laughter and a punch line that never gets old.

When Brit Peter Harris was in town, Dave Haines used to make him repeat the Goldilocks story. "Elroy used to look after me like a prince when I went to America," Peter said. "Really he did. Sometimes he would put me up at his own home. On this particular occasion, I went over for a three-week burst." It was summer, and this time the company put him up in a room in one of the dormitories at nearby Wilmington College. They were up against deadlines, and it would shorten Peter's commute.

"I brought my stuff in, hung up all my clothes, jumped in the car and went to work," Peter said. "After work, I went back, had a shower, then went out for a meal." By the time he finished dinner, it was dark.

"As I walked along the corridor, I had a funny feeling." When he opened the door to his room, he could hear somebody snoring like a buzz saw. "There was a chap asleep on my bed. I just walked a bit farther down the corridor and opened another door." There was an empty bed. Like Goldilocks, he fell fast asleep. "It caused hilarity at the factory the next day."

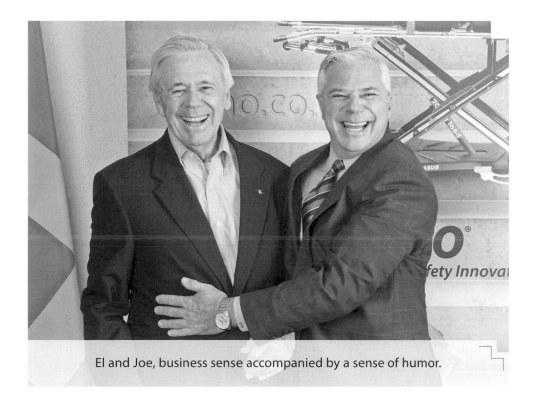

El and Joe, business sense accompanied by a sense of humor.

"You didn't tell him to leave?" somebody asked.

"I just got into another bed, and he was gone in the morning," Peter shrugged.

"The truth was that you estimated the guy was bigger than you," El joked.

Vickie Giannetti, senior executive administrative assistant, wrote an item in the company newsletter, reporting an incident at a sales meeting in 1996 when four Ferno young associates thought they might have beaned the leader of the company during a golf outing. As El finished a hole and was waiting at the next tee, a golf ball burst through some bushes and rolled under the cart. El picked the ball up, staggered through the bushes and threw himself to the ground, holding his head and clutching the ball, right in front of the horrified sales reps.

"I have never seen golfers as scared as those four," reported an employee who'd been riding in El's golf cart. "Especially the one who hit the shot." Years later, Vickie, a gracious and businesslike woman, the gatekeeper to the company's senior executives, chortles gleefully. "Wish I'd been there."

At Ferno, they also love the tale of the trip to a fancy restaurant in Ronnie Hast's hearse. First of all, they have to tell you about Ron Hast, a pretty good story on its own. A high school dropout, he was, according to El, "a learning machine."

Ron, who eventually became publisher of a highly regarded trade publication for funeral directors and co-owner of a successful funeral support company in California, began with a $40 hearse in 1956. He started ferrying flowers from the church to the grave site. Then he started picking up bodies.

"He built his business around our One-Man Cot," El said. Ron began converting Ford station wagons, calling them first-call vehicles or flower cars or junior hearses, adding crinkled vinyl roof coverings and deeply tinted windows for a fraction of the cost of a new Cadillac. Ron Hast and his partner, Allan Abbott, also began working with funeral homes to transport bodies by commercial airlines, designing a Casket Airtray, used for decades throughout the world.

Brass chrome-plated landau bars were "specially made only for us," by Ferno-Washington, according to his posting on the Friends of the Professional Car Society website. During the first year in business, he and Abbott began offering livery service that included both limousine and funeral coaches. They connected with the movie business, supplying funeral cars and props.

When a funeral home was chosen to direct the services of Hollywood royalty, Ron Hast's company would usually be tapped to provide the car and driver. Ron, himself, was a pall bearer at Marilyn Monroe's service at the request of her grieving ex-husband, Joe DiMaggio. The company had supporting roles at the funerals of Natalie Wood, Clark Gable, Jack Benny, Gary Cooper, Ernie Kovacs, Jack Warner, Mario Lanza, David O. Selznick, and Karen Carpenter.

When El met Ron, El said "we hit it off right away," continuing to reconnect at conventions over the years. With a puckish smile and oversized eyeglasses, Ron "was fun, played the piano, and could talk, talk, talk." When Ron's business was in its infancy, "he hired a lot of young people nobody else would take a chance on," El remembered. "He salvaged a lot of lives. Gave them work, made them dress in white shirts and ties. How they appeared and interacted with the funeral directors was basic training, and he set a high standard."

When Brian was a youngster, fragile and suffering from rickets, Ron Hast organized a three-day outing to Disneyland. "He met us with a limo and stuck with us the whole time, pushing Brian's stroller through the park." On another occasion, Ron chartered an amphibious plane to take El and Elaine and the family to Santa Catalina, a rocky island just off the coast of California. "A tiny plane, crummy weather. Elaine was saying her Rosary the whole time." Three days later, an inspector with the FAA fell through the wing during an inspection.

Through the years, El and Ron were sounding boards for each other "for new ideas or ways to improve equipment, methods, and customs in the funeral service industry," El said. "Abbott & Hast was the beta site to field test many products that Ferno developed. We played devil's advocate with each other. He was a good listener, but he never missed an opportunity to challenge the norm in the funeral industry and became an agent of change."

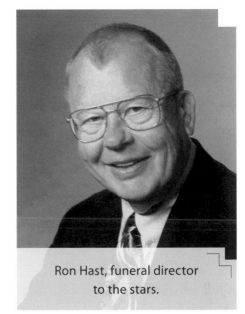

Ron Hast, funeral director to the stars.

In 1973, Abbott & Hast acquired *Mortuary Management* magazine, a monthly trade publication for funeral home owners, staff members, service and supply industries and mortuary students. Curious and observant, Ron noticed that copies of his magazine were scattered around the waiting areas and lobbies of funeral homes. After he took over editorial management, he used scenic pictures and removed cover headlines about embalming and "other issues that could be disquieting to a bereaved family."

However, he didn't mind rattling his primary audience and advertisers with stories inside the magazine about alternative choices for bereaved families, including cremation, and further alienated some readers by his friendship with Jessica Mitford, whose book, *The American Way of Death*, led to Congressional hearings on the funeral industry. Ron, who'd begun leading a series of professional seminars, offered her a place on the dais. "There were a few hecklers," he told an interviewer, but she "did her research and had a lot of good points. We developed a dialog. She was fun, unusual, interesting to be with."

As was Ron.

After a day of schmoozing and seminars at a convention in Las Vegas (which drew not only people from the industry but many spouses as well) Ron Hast gathered about eight people to go out to dinner. The group included El and Elaine, Dick Ferneau, and Gary Hiles. Ron, exuberant as usual, told them it was a fancy place where he knew the maitre d'. Dick, of course, was skeptical. Was it expensive? Dick believed in eating well only if he'd made a lot of sales that day, according to Gary Hiles.

Ron's company exhibited specialty cars at events like this, and many of these vehicles still lumber down the road today, beloved by collectors. El didn't remember exactly which one Ron drove that night, but it was a vehicle that would be hard to ignore. Big and flashy. Ron calmly threw open the oversized doors and herded the dinner party into an enormous black hearse with the signature Abbott & Hast gold numbers on the windshield and a palm leaf appliqué sandblasted on the rear window glass.

Behind the driver's seat, passengers found places on the floor, shielded from prying eyes by elaborate side curtains with a sunburst pattern allowing visibility to the driver but blocking the view from outside. "Off we went," El said. It was... a hearse.

The valet at the upscale restaurant was flustered as the oversized doors flew open and a very-much-alive group scrambled out. "We didn't think that much of it," El said. "But the guy in the parking lot did. His eyes were as big as saucers." He looked behind him at patrons entering the establishment, craning their necks. He glanced down the neat rows of Jaguars and Porches and Mercedes. And in a not-too-quiet voice said, "Where am I supposed to park *this*?"

Having just ended a day surrounded by caskets, embalming fluids, and church trucks, a ride to dinner in a hearse was nothing but appropriate.

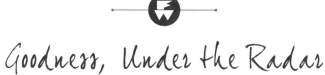

Goodness, Under the Radar

Dick Ferneau was well known to the people who worked at Fayette County Child and Family Services. He was an irregular regular—dropping off checks, cash, and clothing without notice, trying to leave without thanks. They never knew when he might show up. Except at Christmas. They could count on a big pile of toys left at the back door on Christmas Eve.

"Well, for heaven's sake, Dick," El would say, "did you at least save your receipts for taxes?"

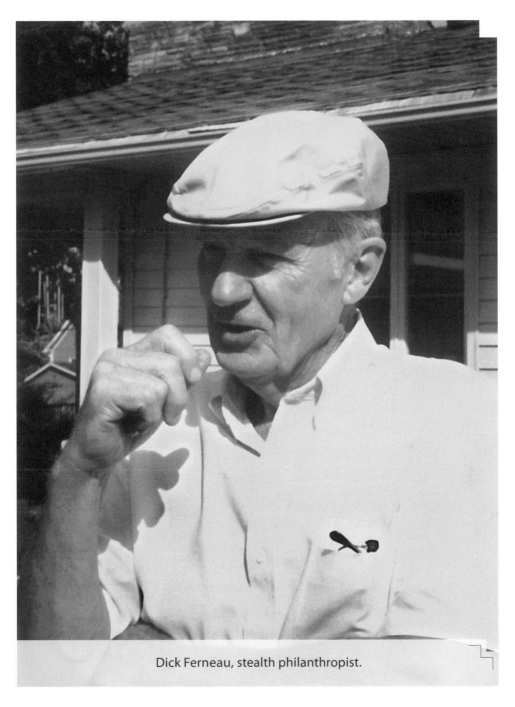

Dick Ferneau, stealth philanthropist.

"Nope."

The Ferno-Washington people, dating back to the co-founders, have the reputation for being good citizens who are more comfortable giving than sticking around to collect the credit.

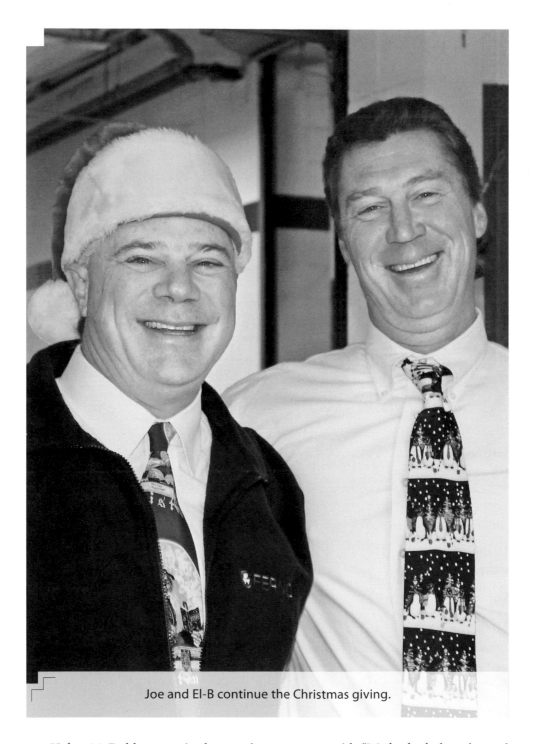

Joe and El-B continue the Christmas giving.

Helen McFadden, a retired executive secretary, said, "We had a lady—she and her husband both worked at Ferno—and she developed cancer. Due to her health and the treatments she was receiving, she couldn't continue on with her job. With the help of Human Resources and everybody working together, she always had a job she could do. She moved to positions she could handle."

Brian Bourgraf discovered there was a concert she particularly wanted to see. Concert tickets mysteriously appeared and a limo showed up to collect her and her husband on the night of the show. "That was marvelous," Helen said. And it just gave you such a good feeling."

During Brian Bourgraf's dialysis treatments, while he was waiting for a new kidney, a Wilmington, Ohio, lawyer and Brian played iPad Scrabble at the hospital. And plotted. They'd gotten to know each other as volunteers at various community fundraisers, including one for a high school music program. The marching band needed carts to roll heavy equipment and instruments onto the field. Brian sent some sketches to the Ferno plant, asking them to make what the students needed. "Don't tell anybody," he told the lawyer. Another time, Brian arranged to deliver waterproof pads Ferno made for stretchers to a Boy Scout troop for use on a camping trip. The pads arrived without a logo, and Brian asked the lawyer not to say where they came from. "Just tell them to go out and be good scouts."

Of course, Brian's assignment as Ferno's corporate affairs coordinator, was to be the charitable face of the company, to serve on boards and committees, to give away money, and to do a lot of that publicly. "It's important for our people to know that we care about their community," El said. So Brian spread Bourgraf Foundation and Ferno money where it was needed, as well as plenty of his own time and money. "I'm guessing he puts in about a hundred hours a month at one charity or another," the lawyer said. And he was not just shaking hands and playing golf. "He was always willing to do the scut work," Sometimes, no matter how hard everybody works, an event just doesn't pull in enough money. Then, he said, he has seen Brian write personal checks.

In a 2014 guest column for the Wilmington *News-Journal*, entitled "Your Life Is Not Your Own," the lawyer wrote about Brian's double kidney transplant and his many gifts of time and money to the community without naming him. "Everybody knew who it was," he said, guessing that Brian's parents had a lot to do with the way he leads his life.

A few years ago, Ellen Coleman was at work in the grinding room when she received a phone call breaking the news that her older brother had been in an accident in Georgia. He was gravely hurt. As she was leaving the plant, Joe

Bourgraf's secretary, Bev Hill, caught up with Ellen and asked if she needed any help getting down there.

"Well, I'm thinking I have to get my other brother...We've got to get down there, but I'm not going to call my sister-in-law, didn't want to ask." When Ellen got to her brother's house an hour or so away, her sister-in-law met her at the door and said, "I just talked to a really nice lady named Bev, and your plane leaves at 4."

The Bourgraf family, according to long-time employee Nancy Keeton, "takes care of a lot of people and a lot of things, and they keep it under wraps." She described helping to form an internal team several years ago. The plan was to "bridge the gap between the production and office workers, help communicate things that were going on as far as business products, a lot of different things. And we just kept growing, and it kind of expanded to community service."

Cathy Williams, a logistics coach at Ferno, connected with several area schools and the Head Start Program. That year, the team raised $1,200 through raffles and donations. At Christmas, they "adopted" a dozen children, buying and wrapping clothing and toys for them. The next year, they added more raffles, then bake sales and canned food drives. They put more kids on the list, branching out beyond Clinton County to Fayette and Highland counties.

Nancy has worked for the company for nearly thirty years, starting part-time in the credit department. "I called people and asked them to pay their bills. That's what my first job was, and I'm now managing International Customer Service. Ferno is my education. That's where I've learned. I got to be a stay-at-home mom until my boys were in high school. And I don't plan to leave until I'm ready to go home and play with great-grandkids or something."

She has been there long enough to have worked with the company's founder. "Mr. Ferneau would slip Cathy checks every year," Nancy said. He'd tell Cathy, "Here. Make sure the kids have enough. Give a little more. You know, do a little more."

Nancy said, "He never wanted thanks for it. He didn't really want a lot of people knowing about it, but he did it every year, and we all knew he would."

They called it Operation Santa, adding food for the children's families. They kicked the fund-raising up a notch, and filled out the paperwork to qualify as non-profit, tax exempt. But the personal involvement stayed the same, and Cathy kept finding kids.

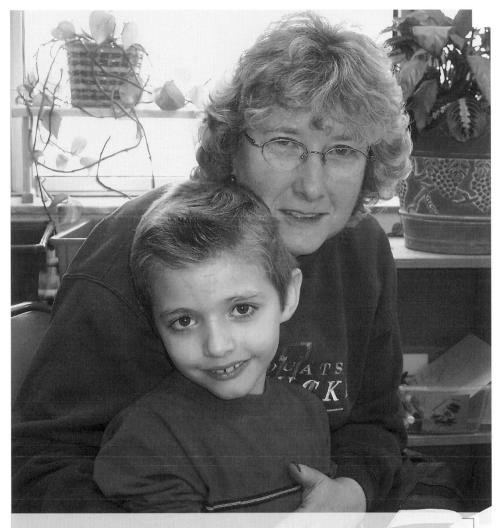

Cathy Williams, in charge of Operation Santa, pictured with her grandson.

A little girl, 4, had never had a doll. So, the team made sure she got one, plus "little pajamas that matched the girl's." And she got a food box. "She was so excited to get Little Vienna sausages, pancake mix, and syrup. She was ecstatic," Nancy marveled, adding, "It makes us all appreciate what we have and makes us aware there are people right next door who don't have. So, we need to look out for each other."

When Cathy Williams retired from Ferno in early 2013 after thirty-seven years with the company, her teammates renamed Operation Santa. Known now as "Cathy's Kids," it most recently "adopted" 103 children and their families. When

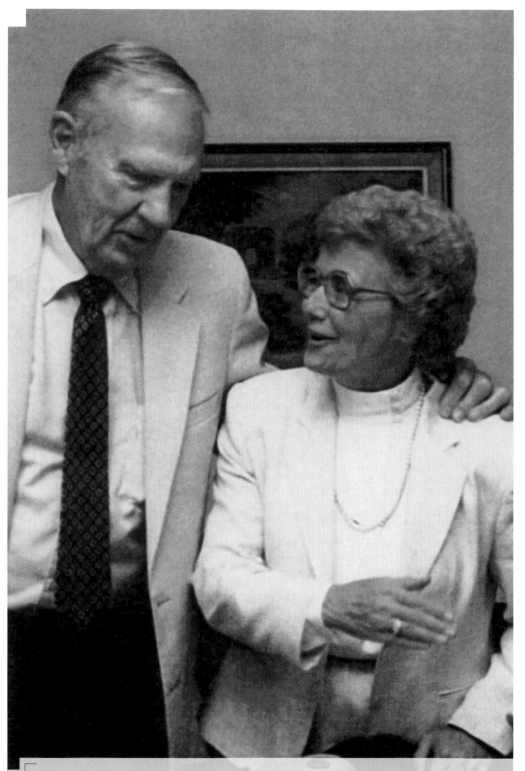

Dick and Helen McFadden.

Cathy Williams lost her battle with cancer in July of 2013, donations poured in from all over the country, and the following year, El Bourgraf presided over the Ferno Community Cookout and Car Show to benefit Cathy's Kids.

The tone of this company is definitely set by its patriarch and reinforced all down the line. In 2014, the University of Cincinnati announced a $1 million endowment from Elaine and El Bourgraf supporting the school's efforts to reach into the new venture business community, bridging the gap between classroom and real world business. Just as he built his world headquarters on a street named for Burt Weil, the man who brought him together with Dick Ferneau, so Elroy Bourgraf honors the place where he collected his business degree. He and Elaine are also stalwart supporters of Children's Hospital and kidney research.

There's a level of decency woven into the company's fabric. "It's who El is and who his sons are," said Dorothy Deaton, Ferno's vice president of legal and regulatory compliance. "They represent the values that we live every day—trust, compassion, doing the right thing. Hard work and getting it done." The lines sometimes blur, she said, between the Bourgraf family and Ferno as a company.

Nancy Keeton said, "That's just what this business is. It's not all products and dollars. We know they have our backs, and we have theirs."

Helen, who retired from Ferno at age 75, remembered her first year at the company. "My husband became very ill and had to be hospitalized in Dayton. Gary Hiles told her to leave her desk and get to the hospital. "That's where you're needed," he said.

Then, she marveled, "Janet Fife, who worked in the International Department, drove me to Dayton, to the hospital. They thought maybe I was too upset to drive. And when we got there, Janet put a wad of money in my hand that I knew had come from Gary and the staff and the Bourgrafs. They took care of you, no matter what. I hadn't been with them very long. But you just don't ever—you never forget that. I was not the only one. They just don't advertise it."

She allowed a small going-away party, but on her last day at Ferno, Helen said, "My goal was to walk out very quietly." She thought she would slip out unnoticed, after hours. The goodbyes, she feared, would be hard to take. "And so I was wrapping it up that evening, when Joe Bourgraf walked down the hall."

And it was Joe, the CEO of a multimillion-dollar global company, who said, "Come on, Helen, I will help you carry your things out to your car."

No Bridges Burned

When the unions came calling in the 1960s, they were disappointed by their reception at the Ferno-Washington plant. It was hard for organizers to convince workers that it would be better for them to take their concerns to a shop steward than to the president of the company who regularly worked shoulder-to-shoulder with them and was a great listener. They knew El Bourgraf. They trusted that he had not only protected their livelihoods but had demonstrated additional respect by sharing what, in some enterprises, is privileged information. Profits, losses, and sales figures were posted on the bulletin board outside the cafeteria for everybody to see.

"We didn't have a layoff until the mid-1970s," El said. Enduring a recession along with the rest of the world, El had to lay off about fifteen employees, by department, by seniority. Gradually, and with great reluctance. Employees had already, literally, seen the writing on the wall.

"We've had about three periods where the economy went down and we had to lay some people off. But most of them got called back to work," said Irvin Pollock, who spent nearly a half century at Ferno and earned a reputation for never being afraid to question his boss about anything, anytime.

"Sometimes we might end up with extra people in some departments, then we'd give them a choice of different jobs or let them take vacation at odd times," El said. Maybe go on vacation early, before they'd technically earned it. But they could catch up later. Employees hankering for, say, a big trip, were allowed to tack on unpaid days to their vacation time, "if they wanted to, if they could afford it." It was their choice, as much as possible. "When times were tough, we kind of danced around, tried to think creatively about keeping people, protecting jobs."

Ferno was the first company in a three-county area to provide a 401(k) pension plan for employees.

Hard to work up real animosity toward management like that.

Dave Haines, who was both labor and management at Ferno during his thirty-one years there, is now a customer. He left to start his own company in 1991 and

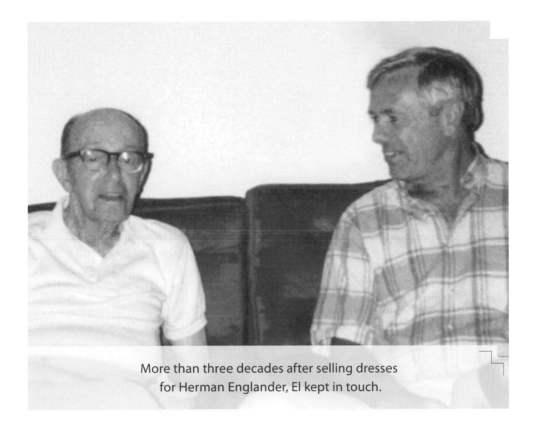

More than three decades after selling dresses
for Herman Englander, El kept in touch.

now is president and CEO of Eastern Area Specialty Transport (EAST), a private
medical transportation service covering Adams, Brown, Clermont, Fayette, Greene,
Highland, Montgomery, Clinton, Ross, and Warren counties.

"We transport people from nursing facilities, long-term health facilities, and
assisted living," Dave said. "If there's an auto accident, they're patched up or
stabilized in a local hospital and then taken to a trauma center for that higher
level of care. Do quite a bit of that." El remembered Dave Haines as "smart, very
mechanical, and good with people."

Clearly proud of his own company, still, Haines said, he wishes he could
duplicate what he experienced at Ferno, "a staff that would support me in a similar
fashion to the people who supported me at Ferno. I was spoiled rotten by their
cooperation and the access to all the things I had. And I miss it. Good place to
work. Good people. Good situation."

Sometimes the situation deteriorated beyond repair. Even among good people.
"I haven't made many enemies through the years," El said. "I never burned any
bridges if I could avoid it." There was a top executive with an impressive resume

who "just didn't cut it." El bumped into him occasionally after the man was fired, and, "We weren't buddy-buddy or anything, but it was cordial." Elroy Bourgraf doesn't have a mean bone in his body, and it shows up in everything he does, including painful business decisions.

Peter Harris, the champion demonstrator of the Ferno Scoop, the border-crossing, and Beatles-singing salesman, was named managing director of Ferno UK in 1985, following his father and sister. In 1993, "Elroy sacked me. He dismissed me," Peter said.

"Once I had to change from being a bit of a pioneer and a creator and come back to be a managing director and more on the direct daily control—scrutiny, what have you—it didn't really suit my personality. And perhaps I could have cooperated a bit more. But I like to do things my own way, and I just made decisions as I had done all my life, and perhaps didn't defer as often as the Americans would have wanted me to before I made those decisions."

Perhaps.

Emergency medical services in the United Kingdom are supervised by the four National Health Services (NHS) of England, Scotland, Wales, and Northern Ireland. The NHS commissioners hold enormous sway over the selection of equipment and care. "Peter had lost some of the ambulance districts. Each had its own politics, and Peter had crossed swords with some of the guys," El said.

John Wilby, who'd joined the ambulance service in 1960, had successfully surfed the politics to become chief ambulance officer in three successive UK services before taking a position in South Africa in 1979 to develop ambulance service there. Then he took over as chief of the Scottish Ambulance Service and then back to London as chief executive of the London Ambulance Service. He was known and respected.

"Even though John had no sales experience, he knew the industry inside out and was on good terms with every single ambulance officer in England. When I terminated Peter, I hired John Wilby. The last thing you want is somebody new to go into a company with a heavy hand. John was a touch of class and a good listener. He didn't have a lot of mechanical aptitude, but he had good people sense."

El's youngest son, El-B, went to England for a year to bridge the gap between Peter and John, whose most immediate contact with Ferno to that point had been as a customer, beginning with the Scoop mailed to him years earlier in a diplomatic pouch by an American friend. "I didn't have much hesitation," John said. "Here was a company that was very much customer oriented, that listened to the customer, that is innovative. I really had every confidence."

John Wilby presided over Ferno UK during its twenty-fifth anniversary year and was at the helm during significant changes. They worked with a relatively new Secretary of State for Health, Virginia Bottomley, and several new products were introduced, including hydrotherapy. The new headquarters in Bradford began to turn out something called the Rescue Rail, designed for the UK to transport patients along railway lines from major disasters.

"My first impression of El was that he was a quiet, unassuming and very gentle man," Wilby said. "He engages people at all levels, and I think that's one of the secrets of Ferno's success—that those at the top understand the problems of those who use the products." That reputation, he said, "permeates throughout the international market. Here is a company that can be trusted and is innovative, develops products jointly with customers."

Those customers, of course, were scattered around the globe. "I never had any trouble working with people in different cultures," El said. It's in his nature "not to try to force our ways on anybody. Sometimes if you pay attention, their way might be better." He learned the art of customer relations, he said, by imitating the way his father dealt with customers those Sundays at the casket company.

CFO Paul Riordan started his career in public accounting, which put him inside a lot of different companies before he settled at Ferno. He said he felt the difference right away. "You keep hearing about the Ferno family. That's really a true belief. You can have disagreements, but at the end of the day, you make a decision and you just move on. Lot of places that doesn't happen. People get angry with each other. There's continuous fighting. But that doesn't happen here. It's just a good working environment. Friendly people, with honest integrity."

A telling measure of El Bourgraf is his tenacity in keeping Dick Ferneau in the Ferno fold. Although he accepted, finally, Dick's desire to leave behind the partnership, he never let his friend, "Henry," disconnect from the company he helped start. El made sure that the "loner" never felt alone, or, worse, unnecessary. Dick stayed on the Ferno payroll for two decades, then when he decided to step back even further, ending his career as a consultant, El sent this letter on June 21, 1997:

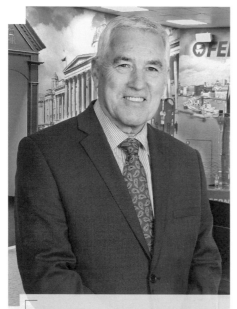

John Wilby was Managing
Director of Ferno UK from 1993–1998.

"Your cohorts had a big team meeting that lasted way too long, but did arrive at a decision to insist that they have a place to leave you messages and information. So even though your office is stripped clean, there will be a few things collecting on the desk for you. Our only hope is that you will stop by at least once or twice a year to pick them up and answer any questions. It will give you a place to hang your hat in case your coat hook rusts out and falls off the wall.

"I've twisted all the necessary arms to assure there is no big shindig scheduled to recognize your change in status. In return, however, we will expect occasional oversight of the various projects going on in R&D. Just want common sense observations and suggestions which everyone around here respects and values."

In December of the same year, El wrote:

"The other week when you and I walked the shop together, I don't know if you noticed the looks we got. Later that day and the next day, at least a dozen people stopped me and commented that it was good to see us walking the shop like we used to do. It was really good for their morale. I'm enclosing your badge, which you must have accidentally dropped in my office. You see, I still want you to pop in once or twice a week, if you can work it in between your yard work and fishing trips. Just take a walk through the shop and try to drag me or Joe along so the troops see you. You don't appreciate how they get a boost just seeing you around, 'cause they like and respect you. You still add a lot of credibility to our organization.

"What I need from my friend is the insight of fifty years experience and lots of common sense hard-ass comments to critique the progress we make on the new Ferno cot. It has got to be a different product, just as the #30 was different from the #54. It will have a different look, and you will not agree with lots of the gyrations we go through to end up with what we hope will be a winner. We want and need your critical insight, and that "we" is more than me. It's a lot of other people who look up to you as the resident ambulance cot genius." And he named a half-dozen employees from the shop and from the office to prove his point.

The "people skills" so prized in modern business manuals were inseparable from El's core values and drew people to him.

Terry Jaques left Ferno, then came back again. Originally an ambulance builder, Les Harris hired him in 1980 as his son, Peter, moved farther afield in Europe. Put in charge of "the whole of the product range and all the market opportunities in England to the south," Terry said it earned him a trip to America, including a reception in the Bourgrafs' cellar and a terrifying ride in El's vintage English taxi. "Unfortunately, one of the things that's very different with a London taxi and American cars is the, um, stick change with a crash gear box," Terry remembered, adding politely that "it was a pity" they did not ask the Brit on board to drive.

Later, he was promoted to the Yorkshire headquarters as a senior sales rep, dealing with ambulance and fire services and funeral directors. In 1990, Terry quit to become a consultant. During the next ten years, he worked for several commercial organizations "that really were competitors in some ways to Ferno," he said. "But I also worked for Northumbria Ambulance Service as director of marketing for two years, which gave me another inside view of the ambulance service." He returned to Ferno in 2000 and stayed in sales with the company for nine years. Ferno was a hard habit to break, he said.

"What comes through very clearly is the passion of the company," he said. "I think they've shaped my personality in a lot of ways. The consideration for other people has come through very strongly from my time with Ferno. They considered me, and they gave me the tools to do the job."

Not long ago, El Bourgraf and Peter Harris met in England, catching up. Peter said after he left Ferno, he "had dealings" with two or three companies. "I never again actually worked for anybody." He went back, he said, to his retailing roots and invested in some outlet stores, and then, "I pursued one of my biggest passions, which is the game of cricket." He became chairman of the local cricket club. "I enjoyed that very much and enjoyed playing as well." Now, firmly, frankly, and happily retired, he and El laughed together, remembering the Goldilocks story.

Recently El sent Peter a collection of puns he'd cadged from the Internet. "I immediately thought of you and your father and your proclivity for the pun.

Many a chuckle we used to have over a sherry before dinner, as both of you used to save them up for our visits. I value and treasure the fond memories of the early days in the UK and then again as you launched our invasion of the mainland markets."

Peter responded: "Ah, yes, those puns. It was and still is a bit of a family tradition, established by my father who would have liked the new additions. It was nice to catch up a little, good to see how Joe has continued the family business. Your story about Joe donating a kidney to Brian was heart warming. You must be very proud. I enjoyed my years with Ferno very much. I am not one to look backwards very often, but that short reunion triggered many memories."

Warmth. Not heat. No bridges burned.

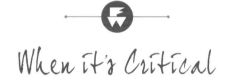

When it's Critical

Pitch-black night sky is pierced by quick strokes of red light and the quiet shattered by a screaming siren. A motorcycle. A curve. A patch of gravel. A skid. The young rider has been flung over his bike into a rocky field. Shadowy figures move toward a figure, crumpled and still. They pluck the body from uneven terrain with a device that parts in the middle to scoop the victim without jostling his back and neck. He's carried swiftly to the waiting ambulance. Within minutes, the siren wails again.

Across the world, on another day at another time, another young man. It was forty-three minutes after kickoff at a soccer match in London. A mid-fielder, Fabrice Muamba, collapsed, falling "like a tree trunk. He didn't put his arms out to break his fall or anything," a bystander said. "He just dropped." A green-clad medical team rushed out with a stretcher. The 23-year-old had suffered a heart attack. He was given CPR, fifteen defibrillator shocks in all—two on the field, one in the tunnel leading out to the ambulance, and twelve on the way to the hospital. A rough trip. One of the paramedics held the waist of the medic, steadying him while he fought to find a vein to receive lifesaving drugs as the rescue vehicle slewed and fishtailed around corners.

Muamba regained consciousness two days later.

"Fabrice had a chance to survive because of all the equipment around the pitch," said another player just after the incident in 2012. "It only takes a few seconds to change a whole life and a whole career." The other player was Petr Cech, a goalkeeper who fractured his head during a game in 2006. He dragged himself off the field and waited for an ambulance. The outcry in the aftermath probably saved Fabrice's life. This time, the equipment and the personnel were standing by.

In both cases, it was Ferno equipment, conceived by Ferno designers and engineers and built by Ferno people who know how it will be used. It's technology and testing and attention to quality details. But Ferno's historic ace in the hole has been relatively low tech: Listening. Respect for the opinions and knowledge and experience of others. No lip service. Putting good information to great use.

No less than Rocco V. Morando, who helped establish EMS in the U.S. and served as the founding executive director for the National Association of Emergency Medical Technicians (NAEMT), remembers both Dick Ferneau and El Bourgraf as allies during the early years. "Ferno worked with us from the beginning," he said. "With guidelines, with standards, with training." Morando was part of the study done by the National Academy of Science on its White Paper report in 1966, which spurred the country to examine emergency medical procedures.

"There was some resistance, but the people at Ferno listened," Morando said. Better still, Ferno "helped spread the word," bringing Rocco Morando in as a speaker at important conventions and industry conferences. More ears. More education.

As EMS systems evolved and medics delivered a higher level of care, more equipment was required inside the ambulance, which led to larger ambulance compartments. The custom built coaches on a Cadillac chassis became obsolete and gave way to the modular box on a truck chassis. Station wagons gave way to small vans. The new ambulances increased the loading height of the ambulance compartment, which made lifting the stretcher into the ambulance more difficult. More women were becoming EMTs just as the population was getting more obese. That, combined with these new load heights, led to a new generation of patient handling cots. They came from Ferno.

In the 1960s, Harvey Hall, now mayor of Bakersfield, California, was just beginning to build the company that would eventually be the largest privately owned medical transportation provider in his state. When El first came calling, Harvey said, "I could tell he had done a lot of background on me. And he was really

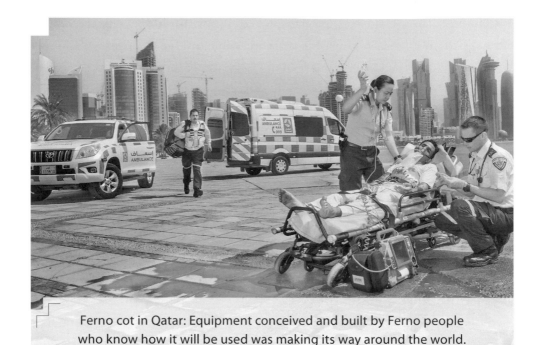

Ferno cot in Qatar: Equipment conceived and built by Ferno people who know how it will be used was making its way around the world.

engaged in what I had to say about my business, like he came to learn." Soon, El was back to talk about Ferno's elevating cots. "It was like the second coming," said Hall, who began his business working in one of his own ambulances with his wife acting as dispatcher from their home. He knew first hand what it was like to wrestle the old stretchers during an emergency call. Back breaking, he told El.

"Listening," El said, "is at the heart of Ferno's culture." As Gary Hiles said, El gets ideas from the guy next to him on the airplane.

Stacy Guerra is a graphic designer, who works on the Ferno catalogs. She's also a volunteer EMT, and her husband is a paramedic and firefighter. Her dad is a fire chief. This is not a pool of information Ferno would be likely to squander. Patients don't come with sturdy, built-in handles. Medics don't always find them where it's easy to place them on cots. Removing patients from cramped spaces often challenges them to use their "inner MacGyver" to figure out a safe solution.

People wander into Stacy's office all the time with questions unrelated to her job description. They know she might be the one to ease an elderly patient into a Ferno EZ Glide stair chair or maybe she'll have her hands on a backboard or need a cervical collar. So, she might be asked, look at this. Would this work better? Be easier to use? More comfortable for the patient? Easier on the paramedics?

Good providers are skilled on a range of patient transport and movement devices, but the places where patients need help are limitless. An EMT might arrive at a call to find a six-foot-plus, 225-pound middle-aged man slumped on the floor of a half bathroom. His wife says he's had "the flu or something" and now is too weak to even crawl.

With barely enough room for two rescuers in the bathroom, they can't position themselves for proper lifting. The room is too small for a backboard or scoop. His size virtually guarantees an injury to the medics or patient if they try to simply drag him from the space. Luckily, he is uninjured, conscious and says he's not in pain. Ferno makes a rescue seat that can be positioned behind the patient, who can then be rolled into a seated position in it. Four built-in handles afford the best possible posture and stance. The rescue duo can move and safely lift his weight and hand him off to others in the hallway.

Another example used in training is a scenario in which a mechanic working under a school bus has been struck by a falling manifold and lies in the bottom of the grease pit. The bus is over the pit on jack stands, all of its wheels removed. Moving the bus is not an option. The only access to the patient is eight steps down a steep, narrow stairway at the far end of the pit.

The patient is unconscious but otherwise stable, with a large lump on the back of his head. There's no room to lift and slide him over the pit's wall to one side or the other. The stairs are the only way out. The head injury, the steep slope, and the tight quarters call for a combination of the redoubtable scoop stretcher, along with a full-body vacuum mattress, which will immobilize the patient without hard-point pressure on his head and conform exactly to his body. The device has built-in restraining straps and six carry handles.

"Ferno makes products," Stacy said, "that let you do your job without worrying about your equipment. You don't have time for your equipment to fail." So many other things her company makes, she said, keep people safe. Things not as noticeable as a stretcher or a backboard. Making a secure clamp for a defibrillator, for instance. "If the ambulance makes a sudden stop," she said, "something like that flying around becomes a deadly weapon."

Enrico Carletti, managing director for Ferno Italy, said his primary goal is to protect the EMS providers, many of whom are volunteers. "Italy has the largest world voluntary association," he said. "What we have pushed in Italy is that Ferno is part of the EMS world. Most of my employees are voluntary EMS guys. In the night, they serve in the ambulances, and days they are working with us. So we know every problem. Absolutely. So, when you talk to the client, he perceives that he is talking with someone like him. It's not we and they. It's one group only."

Gary Hiles recruited Carletti nearly twenty years ago. After an interview in Bologna, the Italian was flown to Wilmington, where, "Gary introduced me to two men in the cafeteria. One of them was Elroy, and one was Dick Ferneau." Meeting them, he said, struggling to express himself, was "like a big hug. Trust, loyalty, available to me, listening to me."

He was shocked. "So that's the bosses talking to you this way? Listening to me?"

It's a big company, said Karen McKenzie, with a small family feeling. Calling herself the "alpha geek," her official title is director of IT. Although employees are scattered across the world and speak different languages, she said, they keep in touch. "We know everybody's names. Anybody can call one of the managing directors from any of the companies, and they can call us. We're all in it together. I know their families. I get prom pictures from Bruce Whitaker up in Canada, and I see pictures of Scott West's children in Australia. And Enrico just had a new grandbaby. So it's a very fun, nice, tight environment for as large as we are."

Beginning at Ferno about twenty years ago as a tech writer, "I didn't really know what I was doing, but my father was a tech writer so I managed to know enough buzz words to get myself in the door," she said. As the networking side of IT was just opening up, she moved over. "The major business system was already here but when we started actually getting PCs on everyone's desk—not just engineering and finance—that was part of my role."

Engaging and direct, she was a natural to bring cyber hesitant newcomers on board, including El. "I call him my poster child. He has large hands, and yet he has one of the smallest little phones, and he can do everything on there. He's very interested in trying new stuff. He's always the first one to say, 'How do I do this? How do I get this working? How can I interface with this piece on that piece?'"

One of the Bourgraf mantras is that they don't expect people to do things they can't or won't do themselves. "El is very receptive, very intelligent, very intuitive. And fun to work with. When he got Bluetooth in his car we sat outside every day for a week, because he kept losing the connection. We'd spend, like, an hour every day. And the next thing you know, we're sitting there jamming to music and waving to people as they come by."

Among other holidays, Ferno employees get Good Friday off. "He used to come in the building and make sure nobody was working," Karen said. "If they were, he'd send them home. I thought that was nice. He's a nice man."

Renee LaPine, who wound up as CEO of a Ferno offshoot, started with the company in the purchasing department when she was eighteen. A co-worker introduced her to a man strolling through the department. "This is El," he said.

"He didn't say Mr. Bourgraf or anything," she said. They chatted briefly, and when he left, Renee turned to her colleague and asked, "Well, who was that?"

"He owns the company," she was told.

"And I thought he just acts like a regular person. He doesn't act like the boss."

Later, the boss would give her a chance to see how she'd act when she was in charge.

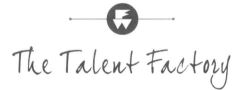

The Talent Factory

When Renee LaPine started work in the purchasing department, there was no computer. "We were doing everything on a posting machine, a card system," she said. "And I was fortunate enough to be part of introducing computer technology into the company." The technology was tested in her department, so she became a de facto cyber pioneer.

The company's first data entry person, she was first to actually run the computer and was front and center of the evolution about to take place. "I feel very blessed, very, very fortunate to have been able to be part of it." Eventually, she moved to customer service, where she helped make that department's technology transition, then she "finally found my home in accounting." That home was productive but, ultimately, temporary. Bigger things were in store for her.

She was smart, talented, and under-educated. People around her at Ferno recognized the first two qualities and helped out with the third. Renee had an opportunity, she said, to learn from effective leadership. The vice president of accounting, she said, "didn't allow for much interaction. We were up there to get

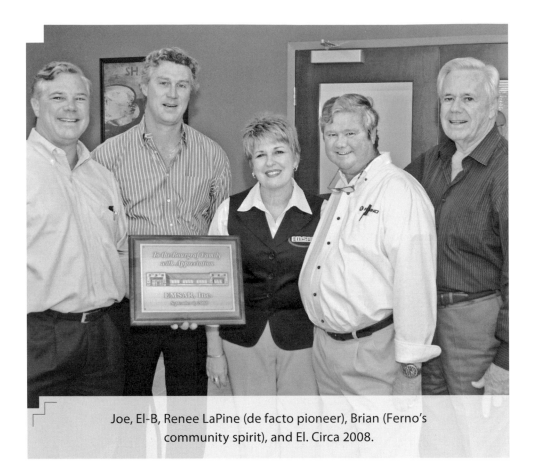

Joe, El-B, Renee LaPine (de facto pioneer), Brian (Ferno's community spirit), and El. Circa 2008.

those books closed and get those reports out so good decisions could be made." Even so, "I would run into El in the shop and just see the respect with which he treated the employees. That resonated with me, and it has been a big part of my development. I saw how he managed himself—with grace and yet, humility. And he was approachable."

After she took a job at Ferno, "it took me probably five years to become a mature employee and understand business practice, but you could tell that El really cared about the employees. I learned that if you treat your employees like family, they will do their best for you."

Experience and observation were fine teachers, but El Bourgraf was a big believer in formal education as well. He pushed his sons toward higher education. And he did the same for his Ferno family. "That has enriched our family culture." Renee's direct supervisor and the controller in the accounting department, Pat Guzzi, had gone back to school herself with help from Ferno and tipped Renee off about the company's education opportunities, encouraging her to pursue her degree.

"If we identified somebody with potential and interest, well, frankly anybody who wanted to go to college, we'd help," El said. "It's a great way to improve the quality of your workforce," El said. Students had to go to classes on their own time—evenings and weekends—and they were required to maintain a B average. Depending on the arrangement, the employee had to agree to stay at the company for a while after finishing school. "A year or two," El said. "There's a buyout plan if they want to leave earlier, but I don't remember anybody ever taking it."

Peter Harris sent Jon Ellis to school on the program, which paid tuition for Ferno employees enrolled at accredited schools abroad as well as area schools including the University of Cincinnati, Wilmington College, Xavier University, and Wright State in programs ranging from engineering to business.

Renee earned a bachelor's degree at Wilmington College. "At that time, Mr. Bourgraf was chairman of the board. So when I graduated from college, the person who handed my degree to me was the person who paid for it." In 1994, she became controller of Ferno's service arm, EMSAR, a franchise company formed in 1993 to support medical device manufacturers. Within two years, she was promoted to vice president of finance and executive vice president before becoming the CEO and president of EMSAR in 1995. "El encourages the entrepreneur in you. He lets you lead the company because he knows you know your business, and he's there as a consultant for you. I just don't think there would be any better situation to have than that."

That too, according to Paul Riordan, is a consistent part of the Ferno culture. "Our guy who ran Ferno UK years ago thought it'd be a good idea to have a power cot, and El said to go ahead and try it. Now that's probably 95 percent of the cots we sell in the UK." Philip Ward, the "guy" who pushed for a power cot and was UK's managing director from 1997 to 2008, said, "Originality sells. It always does." He praised the American parent company for listening to those on the front line of sales and its willingness to customize products to meet disparate needs. "The amount of autonomy allowed in individual markets—it's quite unusual, actually."

Enrico Carletti dared to propose changing the Ferno Scoop, the aging thoroughbred of the equipment stable. "We've made scoops around here forever out

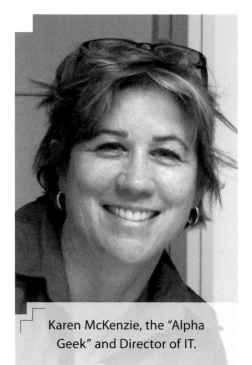

Karen McKenzie, the "Alpha Geek" and Director of IT.

of metal," Riordan laughed. "Enrico made one out of polyethylene." The trifecta, it's durable, colorful, and sleek. "A neat Italian design. We sell thousands of them."

"Power cots, jazzy scoops—the Ferno spirit makes its way into staid finance as well," Riordan said. "I'm not given instructions on what to do every day. It's up to me to come up with what I think is the right thing to do, what's right for the corporation and right for the family."

When Karen McKenzie was climbing the information technology ladder at Ferno, "It was top heavy with men in any type of management role. When I went to conferences, I was one of about three in a hundred. The best thing about working with Ferno is that if you show interest, then you can get in there and get involved. It has nothing to do with your gender or your background. If you have the aptitude and the attitude, you can move forward."

Renee's company, EMSAR, the acronym for Equipment Management Service and Repair, is uniquely independent. Although it's part of the Ferno Group of Companies, it's located off the Ferno main campus, minutes away from Ferno's Wilmington headquarters. It started with Ferno as the number one customer. "We built upon that over the years," she said, "and today we have about 170 technicians nationwide that do the service, repair, and preventive maintenance." EMSAR's broad customer base, which extends across the United States and Canada, includes hospitals, private and municipal EMS service providers, funeral homes, long-term care facilities, dentists, and veterinarians and is the only organization authorized to service both Ferno-Washington and its closest competitor, Stryker.

From her unusual perch as a Ferno "service partner," she said that while the company has grown, "It still has that feel of caring about the employees, caring about customers, and it has a bigger mission than the bottom line. That's when you can really make a difference."

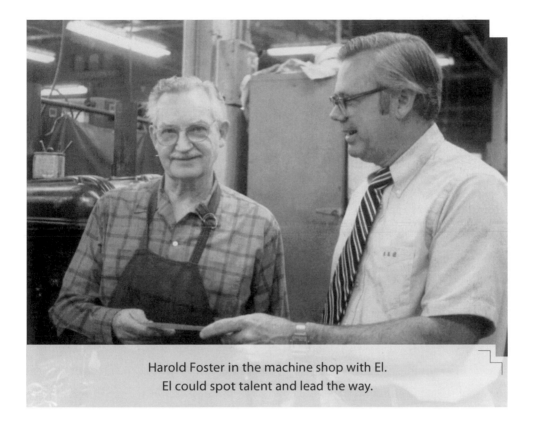

Harold Foster in the machine shop with El.
El could spot talent and lead the way.

In 2014, EMSAR acquired Penn Biomedical Support Inc., headquartered in Blandon, Pennsylvania. "That's going to lead us into product installation in the hospitals. Our hope is to be able to double the size of EMSAR in the next three to five years through either acquisition or organic growth." The new property will provide clinical and communication equipment installation and systems integration support—more computers, more technology in the hands of the person who learned early in her career about embracing cyber tools. EMSAR's CEO also introduced ServiceVue, an equipment management portal tied directly to the system, giving customers access to the service history of all their equipment with a mouse click.

Since her meeting forty years ago with the boss who acted just like a regular person, she learned, "The Bourgrafs are fantastic people to work for. It's the Great American Dream. They helped me with my education. They put me on a path and said 'go for it.' They trust you to make your decisions on a day-to-day basis." Without micromanaging. Spotting talent and nurturing it.

"They let us just spread our wings and fly."

The Ferno Way

Long before "transparency" became a political and corporate buzzword, El made sure everybody in the Ferno family knew what was going on inside the company. At first, of course, the company was small enough for him to stroll through the building and see everybody who worked there every day, hear what they had to say, and maybe cheer lead a little. He could pass along his relentless enthusiasm for the next big idea and solve problems. As the Ferno family grew and he spent more time out of the country, El was determined to keep in touch.

The written word, he said, sometimes expressed his thoughts even better than a conversation.

Notes left on the windshield of Dick Ferneau's car, the letters between partners when the partnership was on the ropes, even notes to his sons. "You have a chance to really think about what you want to say," he said.

So, he started a company newsletter giving voice not only to management but to hundreds of others in the Ferno family. Gary Hiles wrote in 1999, "Secrets are not power. Share information. Value other employees, their thoughts, and their ideas. Mountains can be climbed by establishing a basis of trust and positive reinforcement of consistent communications, follow through and honesty among all employees. I think this just might be the original idea of the Ferno Way."

An aside from El in the same issue praised a Ferno employee who received $100 from the company for kicking the smoking habit for one year. The employee returned the $100 when he started smoking again.

Another item noted that James Combs suggested the handles inside the Aquaciser be changed as the old handles were "ugly" and needed extra adjustments. The new handles saved $300 per unit. This was part of the CRIER program—Cost Recovery is Everyone's Responsibility—headed up by El-B Bourgraf. Eventually, cash rewards and recognition—CRIER awards—were made to people in nearly every department in the company.

Over the years, the newsletter had several iterations, beginning as the Ferno *Scoop*, later the *Ferno Update* and now *The Mobility Connection*. It became the means to "convey a bigger image," El said. "It went out to our workforce—that's who you have to build the family around—then it started going out to our customer base. I wanted them to get a notion of the scope of the company. We are a global company. We want people to know we're doing a big job. We want people in Australia to know we're big in England." Then, with typical humility, he added that it was "an amateur's effort at being a marketing person."

In an early issue, El touched on his concept of the Ferno Way. "The Ferno Way represents the principles and philosophies upon which we conduct business. It is based on truth and common sense. As the needs of business change, we want to face up to them and look for practical solutions. We cannot live with the cliché 'We've always done it that way.' We must search for new, better, and innovative ways to deal with the changing times. I've often said I've got lots of mistakes I've yet to make. Share with me the risk-taking. Let's look out for the customer in the same way we look out for each other."

In a prescient note in 1992, he warned, "The challenge to our country is the forthcoming debate on providing healthcare to the uninsured population. Many political proposals will be heard but I doubt that any solution will result. In the next several years the delivery of medical services will be altered to assure all Americans are guaranteed healthcare. This must be paid for through taxes or redistribution of insurance premiums. Either way, it will affect all of us at Ferno."

He shared his concerns about the cost and complexities of complying with the 1990 Medical Device Act. "Congressional pressure on the FDA will increase the enforcement effort and the burden of our company to comply with the law. The added cost of the red tape will increase our cost of doing business." As usual, he reminded the Ferno family, "We must continue to emphasize good manufacturing practice in our everyday work effort so that we deliver a quality product to our customer. Remember that the customer provides our weekly paycheck."

Earlier that year, El spent nearly a month at a product liability trial at which Ferno was being sued for more than $1 million by the estate of a 72-year-old man who had died seven years earlier. "The EMTs allegedly allowed the Model 30 to fall, causing him injury resulting in his death. The jury ultimately agreed with us that he died of an aneurysm and had been destined to die even before the EMTs arrived on the scene."

As he cooled his heels in the courtroom awaiting the verdict, El ruminated on the seven-year ordeal, the dispute over the design of the time-tested Model 30, and

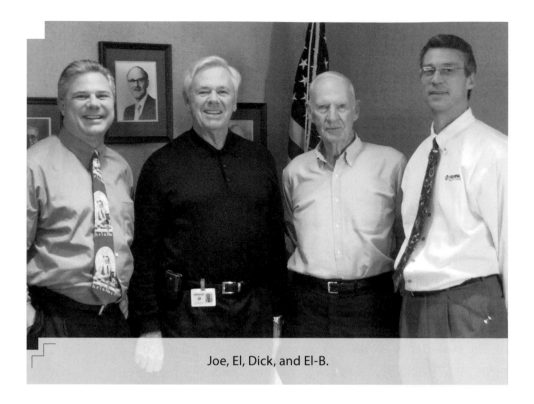

Joe, El, Dick, and El-B.

the process involving thirty-four people at "an unknown cost" in an "overloaded court system," concluding that "the product liability climate in our country adds to the cost of healthcare" and "there is little light at the end of the tunnel."

The only room left for his customary optimism was the country itself. "The jury system works. As I've traveled the world peddling stretchers over the last thirty years, I've never come home and not realized that the United States is still the best place to live and raise a family."

The newsletter evolved into a mishmash of inspirational and pragmatic messages, new employee introductions, opportunities and ideas, recipes and condolences, which like inside jokes offer considerable insight into the character and personality of this company. The financial health of Ferno, posted in sales and inventory reports on the bulletin board outside the cafeteria, were just part of the story El wanted to share with the family, and continued the litany of his product liability travails.

"Every winter when the snow falls and the cold wind blows, it seems the legal system decides to take Ferno to court," he wrote in February of 1995. "Yes, our product liability dilemmas continue, although in most cases we seem to reach a settlement before climbing the courthouse steps. A case involving a wheel that allegedly dropped off an eight-year-old Model 29-M following a haphazard repair job by who-knows-who, resulting in an EMT claiming a back injury. Our chances again look very good for a verdict in our favor, but it will be another expensive victory."

El wrote in April of 1996: "There is nothing that charges my adrenalin as much as listening to a user or buyer of our product come back with a list of complaints and improvements." So, he opened the conversation to include customers.

"The 35A stretcher is a little heavier than we expected," complained a man from an ambulance service in Maryland. "And the person raising and lowering the undercarriage needs to operate the latch as well, so the person holding the end can have a better hold. Also the loading wheels should swivel."

A UK customer noted, "My recommendations for the basket stretcher include: instructions printed more clearly, a picture on stretcher, more detail attaching restraints, hand holds backed up with a carrying strap."

An embalming service in Texas wrote, "We ordered and received our cots. The boxes arrived as if they had been hand-carried across the street."

A New York customer said bluntly, "Prices too high."

Note from El: "We are all winners when controversial subjects get on the table and are open to discussion. It is much better than sifting for an answer in the rumor mill or not knowing both sides of a story. Many questions would be answered if the person asking the question would seek to understand before expecting to be understood. Working together and helping each other can answer a lot of the questions. I encourage everyone to continue to ask the tough questions and, at the same time, make an effort to become part of the answer. That is really the Ferno Way."

The *Update* staff grew to include reporters from every department, yet maintained its nonchalant mix of the personal and professional.

In May of 1999, the big story was an announcement of new branding strategy: Ferno…When It's Critical. "It is no longer a matter of simply building the best products. Buyers are seeking brands that do more than satisfy the 'functionality' of a product. The companies that seek stronger relationships with consumers are growing throughout the United States. These expanding companies strive to create an emotional connection between their companies and the target audience. Our goal is to delve into the hearts and minds of the EMTs. Ferno will become synonymous for action.

"Over the coming months and even years, Ferno will be re-positioned as the only brand that acknowledges, respects and values the 'heroes of the street.' We will create separation from other products by positioning the Ferno brand as the only name to trust when the job is 'really tough.' Product ads will continue to be used to introduce new products. Branding alone will not win the marketing battle. The wise company will prevail through offering powerful brand relationships plus dynamic product offering. Recognizing this opportunity for expansion through the addition of brand-building will assure Ferno a leadership position and a brilliant future."

This corporate announcement was followed by a "Graduate Edition," photos of employees' kids, including one of a young man who caught a twenty-four-inch bass.

A feature entitled "Great Saves" printed a letter from an EMT who used a set of straps off a Ferno cot to pull a friend's car out of the snow. "I strapped one end to my bumper and then the other to her front axle. Then I buckled the clasp. It was a long shot but it worked. Pulled her car out without a hitch. We just unbuckled the clasp and drove to work. Not exactly a great save but a great credit to the quality of your product."

A more dramatic save:

"In sub-zero weather, an EMS team in Skowhegan, Maine, raced to save a 41-year-old man who'd been struck by a swinging beam and was clinging to a catwalk a hundred feet off the ground. "The patient was alert, terrified and complaining of head, neck and back pain. The rescue team huddled and decided to lower him on a basket stretcher using integrated ropes. Nearly two hours after the initial call, the patient was placed in the warm ambulance and was on his way to the hospital."

In his front-page note in another issue, El shared his frustration with foreign knockoffs of Ferno products. "We don't see any one competitor making great inroads, but every one of them is doing some business, which means we are not getting the order. Our product life cycle is rather long and this presents us with a competitive opportunity if we upgrade our present products and innovate our replacements. Let's not forget our original corporate motto was "Good Ideas from Ferno."

Wordlessly, global Ferno was evident in a stream of photographs. Almost every issue pictured international visitors to Wilmington from every corner of the globe.

Occasional references over many years have been made to the Ferno Way, generally described as a system of family values based on integrity, excellence, and innovation. The Ferno Code of Ethics, specific guidelines for all employees, has a whiff of legalese and is explained fully in a policy and procedure manual. But as a rule of thumb, employees are encouraged to ask themselves:

- Is this legal?
- Is this the right thing to do?
- Will this action protect and positively reflect Ferno's ethical reputation?
- How would the results of my actions look in the newspaper or on TV?
- How would my family view my actions?
- Am I being truthful and honest in my actions?

People in this company speak with pride about the products they have built, setting the agenda for an entire industry. Big things. New ideas and products, brilliantly conceived, precisely engineered, rigorously tested. But what they sell is manufactured and sold in an atmosphere of respect and kindness. The blizzard of notes over the years from El, celebrating birthdays and anniversaries and sympathizing with loss. Anonymous generosity. Tactful envelopes of cash in a crisis. A dismissal with civility. Financial disclosures on the bulletin board. Fair pay. Tangible acknowledgment of employee contribution. College tuition. Listening, listening, listening—to the workforce, to the customers, and to the community.

"You can put a lot of big words around it," Joe said, "but at the end of the day our time on this earth is short, and if we can help other human beings, I think that's the Ferno Way." It is not a call to action. It does not set a direction so much as describe and reinforce an existing way of doing business, a solid and long-standing foundation.

"We have some talented people, some veterans with a world of experience, a willingness to continue to invest and the confidence that we are not afraid to make a change."

6

Critical Moves

Reclaiming Lost Ground

El Bourgraf had made a mistake. Considering the complexity of his business and his years of solo leadership, he hadn't made many. But this one was a whopper.

In 1985, El and Elaine bought a place in Naples, Florida, on the Gulf Coast, a warm weather getaway. With its seven miles of white sand beaches, balmy weather, golf, fine restaurants, upscale shops, and unusual variety of cultural attractions, Naples was sometimes a hard place to leave. It became a favorite spot to entertain friends from the international Ferno family, such as the Harrises from England and the Larsens from Norway. Over the next decade, the Florida getaways were extended, and El started thinking about stepping back from his day-to-day responsibilities. Ferno needed to continue forward, but El was ready to put somebody else in the driver's seat.

A candidate presented himself. An executive at a highly regarded company in Cincinnati, he had gone to good schools and had pumped some additional Ivy League training into his resume. El knew him socially and was impressed. "I heard a lot of highfaluting words executives are supposed to use," El said. "And I just didn't vet him, didn't dig deep enough. I held on for about a year. It's difficult to recognize your own mistakes, and I learned it's dangerous to both parties to hire a friend at a high level."

Bernie Zoldak was El's mulligan. He would not get another.

The new hire "wasn't building relationships inside or outside the plant." He wasn't meeting his own financial projections. "The company was not growing. In fact, Ferno was losing ground. It just wasn't working," El said. "When I terminated him, I did it verbally and followed it up with a letter, then put a concise message on the bulletin board. I didn't trash him." El took a deep breath. He postponed his plan to ease out of the company and came back to his desk to repair the damage.

He found a new ally waiting for him. "Before I reported to work for my first day," Ron Beymer said, "I found out that my new boss had been fired." Handsome and trim with white hair and a good smile, Ron, then VP of engineering, received new directions. He was to put some structure back into the company. "The culture had gone awry," Ron said. "It was right after Stryker had gotten into the market, so it was a very interesting time."

El told Ron they needed to improve the quality of the product, get the customer focus back, and get personal responsibility back in the business. El's ambition was to not only reclaim lost ground but to put the company on a new trajectory of growth. "We had to develop some structures to deliver this," Ron said.

Both Ron, hired to head up engineering, and CFO Paul Riordan had come from Belcan Corporation, a Cincinnati engineering and consulting company. Graduates of the Covey leadership program, they agreed that the principles were consistent with Ferno's. Based on Stephen Covey's wildly popular book, *The Seven Habits of Highly Effective People*, first published in 1989, the program's clients eventually included about seventy-five percent of Fortune 500 companies and at least three dozen heads of state. Paul and Ron involved El-B and Ferno's facility manager Larry Newberry, then the Covey leadership training was offered first to Ferno's leadership, then to employees throughout the company. "If they were willing to do the work, El would pay for it."

The approach, called "the Character Ethic," was presented in a series of habits progressing from dependence to interdependence. "Team and process training. How to make teams work. Setting goals. It seemed like a perfect fit," Ron said. Hired originally as vice president of engineering, Ron was promoted six years later to executive vice president. In between, he guesses he sent about 150 Ferno employees through the Covey program. The message was "Good enough isn't." In 1997, he helped create an incentive plan in Wilmington, based on group performance. Managing directors around the globe were put on a similar incentive plan based on the results of their own divisions.

"We tried to teach people that everything they do can have an impact on the whole group," he said. All employees at Ferno get a cash gift at Thanksgiving based on their years of service. The bonus they get at the end of the year is not a gift, but a reward for performance, an incentive based on the company's profitability that year. "You matter" is the message.

"El definitely pulled things back together," Ron said. "He started a major turnaround. He helped us focus." But the company's CEO still had one foot out of town.

Dick Ferneau was worried, which was his customary state of mind. But this time it wasn't unions or balky church truck wheels that agitated him. For maybe the first time since the Bomgardners had abandoned their stretcher business, he was

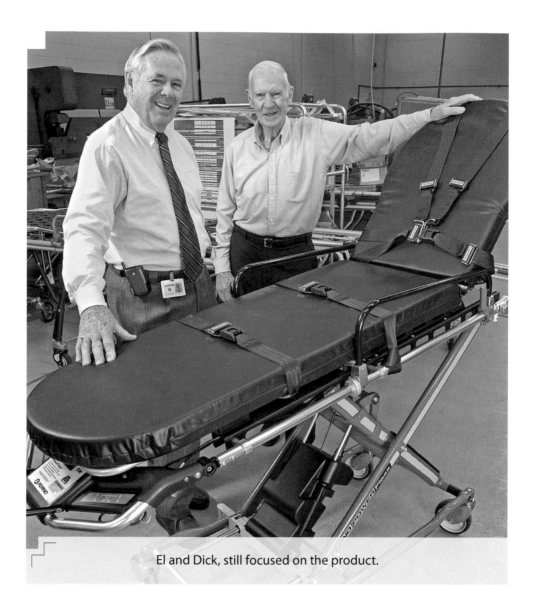

El and Dick, still focused on the product.

seriously apprehensive about competition. Stryker, the medical device behemoth, had lumbered squarely into Ferno's path.

Incorporated in 1946 by Homer Stryker, an orthopedic surgeon and inventor, the company's first patent was for the oscillating saw used to remove plaster casts, the forerunner to a broad line of surgical instruments. A decade later, Dr. Stryker invented the turning hospital bed, which looked like a small Ferris wheel and allowed immobile patients to be re-positioned, helping to prevent bedsores and easing the lifting chore for medical workers. Later came an oscillating bone saw used during chest surgery and a rubber heel for walking casts.

The Orthopedic Frame Company, which posed earnings of $1 million in 1958, became Stryker International, Inc. in 1964. Homer's son, Lee, took over the company in 1969 and began to develop sales forces in Canada and overseas in 1972. "Stryker tried to buy us several times over the years," El remembered. "We decided to work together instead. Lee and I had kind of a handshake deal. "El said he'd stay out of the hospital if Stryker would stay out of the ambulance. For the next half dozen years or so, the two companies cooperated. Stryker built the undercarriage of its hospital stretchers and Ferno supplied the tops—the patient surface. "Many of the features we'd developed for our ambulance stretchers were incorporated into Stryker's products," El said, "Ferno was instrumental in developing the Stryker hospital stretcher."

When Lee Stryker died in an airplane crash in 1976, the handshake deal died with him.

By 1980, Stryker International was being traded publicly and the company was selling stretchers manufactured in-house, including tops. In 1994, Stryker heralded its EMS Cot launch: "With their distinctive yellow and black design, the first model helps Stryker gain quick access and success in its first non-hospital market."

El dismissed the cot, calling it "our product painted a different color." As far as the EMS market was concerned, El considered Stryker a johnny-come-lately and a copycat. As Stryker was splashing around yellow paint and logos, El clung to the clean look of aluminum and the Ferno name discreetly imprinted on a little tag along with the model and series numbers. "I thought it looked more professional," he said.

"The marketing types started bugging me about getting the name where people could see it." Color began to make its way into the Ferno product lineup, and "I became in total agreement that we should put our name everywhere we could blast it."

Following a conversation with Dick Ferneau in 1997, El tried to reassure his former partner, writing, "We ended up the last fiscal year with about $3 million profit, reduced the bank debt by close to $6 million, and I actually had some fun again. Believe it or not, I think I see light at the end of the tunnel. I say this being fully aware of the Stryker cot and more aware of the threatening competition in Europe."

He allowed that Stryker "has done a hell of a good job, but it took them over two years and several million dollars of investment." In his view, Stryker threw good R&D money away "trying to improve our product. They made a lot of the same mistakes we had committed." Still confident of Ferno's superior products, ideas, and organization, he conceded that compared to vanquished rivals like the Bomgardners, Stryker had more patience and a lot more money.

"They are still giving away a lot of their cots just to get people to use them and only have one product, with nothing to compete with the #93, or the #28 Ferno-Flex cot, or the couple of dozen other items we have in our bag. Our distribution system is still much stronger and getting stronger." El had mended the internal and external fences that had splintered during the failed executive's reign. Ferno had history, momentum, and relationships.

"It's a big country and bigger world, and they can't take it all away overnight. Not to say they will not last and will not take some market share. After all the product evolution Stryker has been through, all they have is a copy of the Ferno #35 with a few gimmicks. Not to say it isn't good and we should not react immediately, which we are doing."

Just as when he began his sweep across Europe with the Harrises, El had faith in research and development and in engineering the product to suit specific customer's needs. "Our next generation cot is already in the incubator. They will not be the lead dog and will continue in the position where the view never changes. We will be proactive with features like the new locking system, like the telescoping handles for ergonomic carrying. We have some talented people, some veterans with a world of experience, a willingness to continue to invest and the confidence that we are not afraid to make a change."

All that said and sincerely meant, El realized, it was not a cakewalk. Not by a long shot. "We were getting to the size when we needed additional management, ready to go to another plateau." He, himself, had to have the confidence to make a big change.

"Just like when Dick knew he had to leave, I was getting to the same point. I had too many balls in the air. I needed help. Somebody with authority needed to be there all the time, not just thinking about it, but actually doing it." Picking up the pieces after the departure of his top exec, turning up the heat on his remaining team, and reinvigorating the company's mission, El admitted that he was still drawn to his Florida retreat and no longer had the appetite for day-to-day operations. He conceded, "You just can't run a business from a distance."

Gary Hiles finally confronted his mentor, respectfully but honestly, the way he'd been taught. The answer is right in front of you, Gary told him.

Joe.

A Healthy Exchange

The oldest Bourgraf son had been working at Ferno since 1991. His title? "Well, we have never been much for titles," El said. But, of course, he had the ultimate title. Bourgraf. It could be a double-edged sword. Much was expected and Joe was following in revered moccasins. Of course, his Ferno education began long before he joined the company. It wasn't just Saturdays at the plant, finding wheels, casters, and shanks to assemble. The business day didn't end at 5 o'clock and didn't always take place at the Ferno plant. The Bourgrafs hosted a nearly constant stream of international visitors at their home.

"With my parents," Joe said, "you saw them work very hard, but you also saw them enjoy the international relationships my father was establishing. We'd have people at our house from all around the world." The oldest Bourgraf son was expected to put on a coat and tie and participate at the dinner table. The boy who taught Swedish visitor Hans Andersson how to throw a spiral pass was learning something in return. "It gave me such diversity and vision as to what else was going on in the world beyond Greenfield and Cincinnati."

"I always suspected Joe might come to work at Ferno, but it had to be his call," El said. And he had to be prepared. The Ferno family was loyal, but they would look hard at the next generation of leadership.

"As a kid growing up, the expectation generally was that you had to get a couple years outside under your belt. College was expected, getting through a university with a parchment paper and having the basis. But after that, to get some real world experience. And, we had to bring value to the business," Joe said.

His talent and interest drew him into information technology. When he joined Sperry after college—it was Sperry Univac at that time—he was with the company through its merger with Burroughs, which became Unisys. "A unique opportunity," Joe called it, "because you got to play in very large accounts and work with technology that controlled grand systems—airlines, banks, governmental operations."

Joe and his wife, Lisa, had worked for several years in Los Angeles before Joe's work with Unisys took them to Houston, where he led the company's software redesign for Continental and Eastern Airlines. Lisa had found an executive position with Continental in the financial department. But their family was growing and "we decided we'd like to get back up to where the grandparents were." Lisa VanAtta Bourgraf, too, had significant Midwestern roots. A Miami University graduate, Lisa came from a family of funeral directors dating back to the early 1900s.

During the Christmas holidays in 1990, El and Joe began talking seriously about his joining the company. Up until then, Joe had shown little inclination to follow a career at Ferno. In 1984, he wrote, "When I look at what it has to offer, it's great. Recession proof (to a point), sole source marketplace, diversified in the health care industry, a solid and committed work force, along with many other aspects which produce a favorable organization. The fact still remains that I'm not sure I want to end up in the business. Being even more candid would direct me to say I could never work for you, but maybe *with* you."

Joe and his father both have joked that "we couldn't agree on how to take out the trash."

A few years later, El invited Joe to attend a sales meeting. "I was glad you came back and hope you got something out of it. I couldn't spend a lot of time with you as I didn't want the guys to read something into it. It did give many of them a chance to meet you again and realize you've got your head screwed on right," El wrote.

As Joe continued to climb up the corporate ladder of a company across the country, El was patient. "It's hard at times to keep your mouth shut and just listen, but it always pays off in the long run," he said. "It's kind of like a golf swing. God give me the strength to hit the ball easy."

"I was a very strong willed person," Joe said, "and it just didn't feel right or fit me at the time. My father was a very strong believer that you need to go out, cut your own mustard, earn your own dollar, and gain knowledge outside of what we did as a family or in the family business. Quite frankly, it was liberating. It was a freedom that you ended up going out and finding your own way."

Meanwhile, El had toyed with the idea of selling the company and even poked around at the notion of taking it public. But Joe coming home to work at Ferno and bringing grandchildren and his wife to Ohio? Maybe taking over someday? This was better. Much better. El used to kid his oldest son, saying that if Joe ever decided he wanted to work for Ferno, he just hoped he could afford

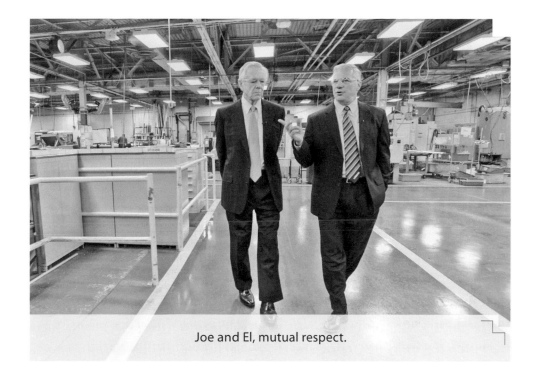
Joe and El, mutual respect.

him. When Joe and Lisa decided to make the move back home to Cincinnati, technically Ferno *couldn't* afford him. Joe took a $30,000 annual cut in pay to come home.

"I'm a very proud dad for what you have already accomplished. The success you have had swells my chest, and I have been known to brag about it. You have survived in a very competitive business and done it with style," El said, sounding very much like his own father decades earlier. The patriarch was eager to see what his son could accomplish at Ferno.

"Joe was good at relating to people," El said. "He had a lot of the same strengths as Peter Harris in that way. He started building relationships in the plant, developing confidence." He shored up international relationships as well, making the rounds of operating entities.

Behind the scenes, father and son often butted heads. Joe nearly quit at least twice. Their exchanges were frank, sometimes funny, sometimes grumpy, and although their correspondence consisted of letters or faxes or e-mails instead of notes left under the windshield wiper of a car or in a toolbox, the tone is reminiscent of the communication between Ish and Henry during Ferno's formative years. Fond, respectful. Tackling problems head on.

In an almost-resignation letter—"I'm tired and frustrated and looking at alternative directions"—Joe ends with, "I will always love you and respect what you have done and stand for."

El advised: "You are the Ferno of the future and need to play the part, only play it the Burt Weil way. You have the tools, smarts, and ability, and need to be perceived that way. Burt had more ideas in a day than I had in a month, but to hear him talk, everybody else had all the ideas, which just happened to coincide with his."

And, "You are more aggressive and in the new competitive environment, it could well be exactly what Ferno needs."

Just because Joe came to work at Ferno didn't mean that getting the top job was a foregone conclusion, a slam dunk, in El's words. "Joe's very much a marketing guy, sales driven," El-B said. "Dad saw Brian in human resources, community services, and things like that. For myself, I was very much into putting things together and running them, and figuring out how to make it better. So, that was sort of the vision that my father had. And, that's pretty much where it all landed. I mean we all landed in those areas."

So, according to the plan, Joe earned his way through marketing, research and development, international development, manufacturing, and strategic planning. Instrumental in establishing Ferno subsidiaries in Slovakia and British Columbia, he also led Ferno through the acquisition and integration of Ferno product lines and subsidiaries in England, Ireland, Scandinavia, and Germany, as well as in the U.S. By the time Ron Beymer reported to work, Joe was managing the emergency division of Ferno. "That allowed me then to get a full understanding of both the international and the domestic customer base, what our product is for and how it all came together to serve our customers."

And, also according to the plan, Joe brought an outside perspective, learned from cutting his own mustard. "They say with each generation, you've got to put a mark on the business," he said. The year Joe joined the company, Ferno had two personal computers and one mainframe. "Ferno was not quite into the technology age. I started to push on that part of the business, asking about our longer term strategies associated with information technology and how it can support and grow the business."

Joe knew the industry and Ferno's place in it. He had forged relationships on his own hook. He had ideas and vision. He is ready, Gary Hiles told El firmly.

And El listened.

The Writing on the Wall

El and Joe made a big production out of the change in leadership. They had to. The elder Bourgraf would still be a vigorous and visible part of the company he founded. As chairman, he said he'd be looking at the company "from 30,000 feet." Joe, as Ferno's president, would be in charge at ground level. Joe moved into El's office. "It was very symbolic," Joe said. "Important psychologically." Joe made an appointment with his father whom he never called "Dad" around the plant or at business meetings around the globe. Calling his father Elroy or, sometimes El, was a mark of respect and a signal of independence as well.

Right on time for the "appointment" in 1999, taking over that office, that desk, Joe thought about the past, "the time and effort he put into building the organization." And he was keenly aware of those who helped. "Dad always used to say that with each employee there was a family. So the decisions you make affect more than just the number of employees that we may have. It's a tremendous responsibility, so I don't take any of it lightly."

He absorbed it all, while deciding how he would build his own leadership. He drew, he said, on the examples of his mother, "who was active in philanthropic organizations." He saw her can-do attitude early and often as she organized a newcomer's club in Greenfield and later put her charm to work on good causes in Cincinnati. He admired his maternal grandparents' work ethic and watching them "interact with their customers within the environment of an open air produce market." He had high regard and fond memories of Burt Weil. "I was blessed to have him in my life." He listened to Uncle Dick Ferneau and watched him scribble and doodle, saw him turn his rough drawings into new products.

Sometimes Dick would take the rough design, sketched on the back of an envelope or even a cocktail napkin, into the shop and finish by borrowing parts from older products, sometimes re-working a mechanical fixture, the support that holds work steady, transferring the skill of the toolmaker to the worker and to the end product.

Joe is quick to credit the human fixtures in his life.

Joe said of his father: "He has great experience and knowledge of how the organization was built and how it served the customers for many years. There are certain characteristics that you embed throughout the organization and you believe in without compromise. Humility is definitely one of those. It's really simple. I'll never ask anybody in this organization to do anything that I wouldn't do."

During their time together at the company from 1991 until the end of the century, when El stepped aside, father and son built on their mutual respect. "Joe explained the ambulance to me," El said once. "I never got beyond the equipment."

"We bounce things off each other," Joe said. "You listen, and most of the time we either meet in the middle or convince one or the other. At other times, we don't even need to talk about it. We kind of look at each other and know."

Elroy moved his belongings to a nice, but lesser space, carrying personal photographs and the only award he'd ever displayed, Outstanding Business Achievement Award bestowed in 1997 to Elroy Bourgraf by the University of Cincinnati Carl H. Lindner College of Business. "Carl Lindner, to me, was the ultimate entrepreneur. He started with a tiny little ice cream store, and the next thing you know he's a billionaire."

At his death in 2011, Lindner was chairman of American Financial, a Cincinnati-based financial holding company that had more than $17 billion in assets. Impressive, of course. But El was most taken with "the total person" of the business magnate with whom he said he had a nodding acquaintance. "He was a philanthropist who put his money where he could make a difference. A lot of what he did was anonymous. And he looked out for the people who worked for him."

The man El called Billy Keating "gave me a lot of insight into Carl." William J. Keating Jr., an influential Cincinnati attorney with the firm of Keating Muething & Klekamp, also handled some of Lindner's business and was among El's most cherished friends and trusted advisers. "He's almost like another son to me. I think I was Bill's first corporate client," El said. "We had good vibes. He's the best listener I've ever known." Their business friendship was nurtured on the humid sidelines of swim meets when El-B competed on the St. Xavier High School swim team.

Being the loyal parent of a competitive swimmer is not for sissies. Elaine got up every morning at 5:30 to get El-B to the pool in time for practice. Then she and El sat through two hours of competition at each meet for, as El said ruefully, "twenty-five seconds of watching your kid in the water."

The Keating Natatorium at St. X was built in 1969 by Bill Jr.'s father and uncle. Sportswriters called it a "Jewel of a Pool." Bill Keating Jr., who was a standout swimmer on the St. X team, continued his allegiance to his family's legacy and his own high school team. El had plenty of time to get to know the young man who showed up at meets, possibly St. Xavier High School's most ardent fan and cheerleader.

For years, El had relied on attorney Lewis Levy. "He was Burt Weil's lawyer, and he wound up representing all of us—Dick, Burt, Ferno and me. It was very unusual, but all of us trusted Lewis's judgment. He was more of a mediator than a negotiator." When Levy retired, El began seeking advice from his poolside friend.

Although El had consulted various other lawyers for advice about patents and labor law, "Bernie and I knew we needed a corporate attorney. It was nothing epic. Initially, it was little stuff. When we needed Bill, he was there." Effusive with praise for the attorney, El says Keating has been central to his and Elaine's estate planning as well as a sounding board and executor of many of Ferno's most important business moves. "Any legal decision we make, Bill is part of it."

The two talk frequently. "If I call him at 6:30 in the morning, he's there. "El is an avid follower of Keating's internet blog, and the two also have worked together on various committees and boards to benefit their mutual alma mater, the University of Cincinnati. "So, the Lindner Award was special to me for many reasons," El said. His other awards, and there are several, hang in the private bathroom of the president's office.

After the ceremonial moving day, El puttered around his new office, unpacking boxes and purposely staying out of the way. "We swapped offices," El said, "to send a message to everybody in the plant that Joe was the boss."

Joe celebrated by working harder than ever.

"There's an announcement, then there's this symbolic physical aspect. But at the end of the day, doing that transition is being present, active in every aspect of the business, and having that passion to getting it done, keeping the organization growing. People know that you're either engaged or you're not. It requires an energy level that everybody can rally around. So president may be a great title, but it's the effort and the dedication behind it that make it real."

And when somebody, maybe an old hand from the shop, maybe a manager, would come to El griping about something or with an idea requiring a decision,

El would point them to the man in charge, making it clear that Joe's new title was not ceremonial. He never permitted an end run around the new president and any advice El had for his son was delivered privately. He displayed utter confidence in Joe's abilities.

"It was an evolution," El said. "I have slowly extricated myself from any active involvement in the plant. When Joe took over, I was still his shadow, ears turned on, still going to work. At first five days a week, then four." Then El started spending chunks of the winter in Naples, coming back once a month for a week, November through May." If he was in Cincinnati, he turned off his cell phone on Wednesdays for a few hours of gin rummy with pals. Now he spends most of the winter with Elaine in Naples.

He joins the Ferno management team every Monday, usually electronically. "I still visit Wilmington, but it's more PR than management. I'm still close with the people I know. I still listen and observe, but I limit my comments to Joe alone." Joe had bounced in and out of the business from childhood and had served his time in the grinding room. The worldwide Ferno family knew him and had seen that, as El said, "His head was screwed on right."

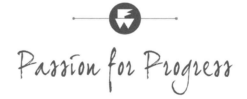

Passion for Progress

Joe gathered the reins and galloped toward the future. His first priority was international growth. "We had a dominant position in the U.S. market and in a number of markets around the world. It allowed me to take a step back and say, 'where do we need to be focusing?'" Where in the world will Ferno go next? There's one simple test, he said. "Look at the value of life, how it's viewed by the government, by the people who live there. A country is ready for our products when you see growing respect for human life."

He set his immediate sights on Poland, Slovakia, the Czech Republic, Hungary, and Estonia. Silvia Vancova, with Ferno since 2001 and now managing director of Ferno Slovakia, said, "What Ferno brought was a different approach to people, values spread through companies as a family. We can exchange experience, share ideas, and it's not just a small pool. It is quite a big company, but it's under one Ferno roof."

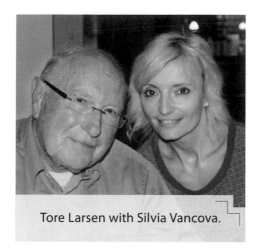

Tore Larsen with Silvia Vancova.

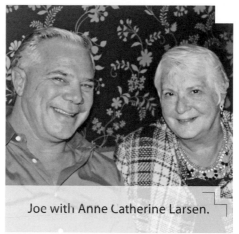

Joe with Anne Catherine Larsen.

Ferno Slovakia, which has a strong R&D component, manufactures and services Ferno products for Central and Eastern European distribution. "Our main focus," the managing director says, "is to deliver and produce products for Ferno group companies. We are growing fast, and we try to absorb more responsibilities for service activities in Central and Eastern Europe. Our boys are working to try to turn Joe's dreams into physical products."

Simon Zerihun of Ferno Middle East, who joined the company in 1988, is responsible for sales in Saudi Arabia, Kuwait, Bahrain, Qatar, Oman, and the United Arab Emirates. Peter Peemans, who joined the company two years later, "looks after" western Europe, and North Africa, as well as Lebanon, Jordan, Syria and Egypt. Peemans praised the "really big difference between Ferno and other companies—not telling you what to do but making you want to do something."

In a letter to Joe from El on April 24 of 2000, El wrote, "You are establishing your own style, but doing it within the principles of the Ferno Way. Change was and is needed. The real challenge is to find how to best benefit from the wealth of experience and history without retarding needed change. You are slowly getting a good team together, and sometimes it can't be rushed."

Joe found a key member of his team in the UK, Philip Ward, who revitalized that division. Named managing director in 1997, Ward said. "Ferno had a very profitable market but they had it all to themselves and competition decided they would come in and take a bite." Sales were soft, plus the Brit bumped up against Ferno's chronic challenge: The product was strong, well made, and *lasted a long time*. He estimated there were about 5,000 ambulances in the UK, and although

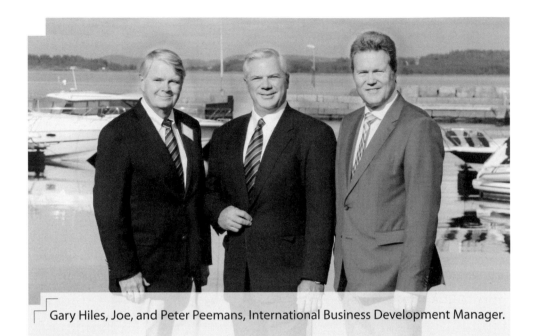

Gary Hiles, Joe, and Peter Peemans, International Business Development Manager.

most of them were equipped with a Ferno cot, the fleet was never going to grow appreciably. "They'd replace a vehicle every few years and just move the old Ferno cot into the new ambulance."

The new managing director organized a contest to find the oldest Ferno cot in operation, and, although he was slightly horrified, he awarded a magnum of champagne to the sales manager who found it. The cot was twenty-eight years old and still in service. "We asked for it back and gave them a brand new one. We wanted to see what this thing was like. It was dangerous. The top wasn't sitting correctly on the bottom. It was twisted. It was worn, but as far as they were concerned, it still worked. They were changing their ambulances every five to seven years. When a new vehicle arrived, they looked in the old vehicle and said, 'Oh, that cot's fantastic. We'll put it in the new one.' And off they went."

Ward realized he had to take control of the product's life cycle to determine when the cot was no longer safe to use. "So we designed, invented, and patented a little device called the Tracker, which fitted to every cot that we produced. It actually recorded the number of times the cot moved up and down or in and out of the vehicle." He created a service division to follow up.

Next, he began talking to his biggest customer about their biggest problem. The UK's National Health Service (NHS) employs 500,000 people, "funded by all of us taxpayers," he said, "and it's heavily unionized. The biggest, biggest problem they had, both in the pre-hospital market and in the in-hospital market, was back injury."

Included in the casualties were paramedics, technicians, and nurses and compounding the problem was the ever-increasing girth of their patients. "The occurrence of injury, particularly to pre-hospital paramedic staff, was unbelievable," he said. When his staff dug into the history of back injuries in that population, they found, "When a paramedic was told that he would have

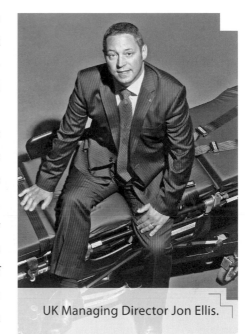

UK Managing Director Jon Ellis.

to give up that job thirty or forty years ago, that guy would retire gracefully, take his gold watch and wish everybody good luck."

The result of union intervention, he said, was that injured workers were spurning the gold watch and graceful retreat, choosing instead to demand compensation from the NHS. When Philip Ward mounted the research project in the late 1990s, he found that sixty-two percent of paramedics in the UK were not reaching retirement age purely through back injury.

"When I first got that statistic, I said, 'You mean 6.2 percent?' No. It was sixty-two percent. So that presented an enormous opportunity, which I grabbed." He set about eliminating two words from the work life of paramedics and ambulance technicians—lift and bend. The idea, he said, came from watching a muffler repair shop. "One man with the aid of a small piece of equipment can lift a two-ton car off the ground. Simple hydraulics. We took those ideas and built them into our designs."

He had some initial difficulty. "The UK market is so different from many markets around the world. Yes, everybody is still collecting a patient and taking them to a place of safety or a hospital, but you would be amazed at the national, regional and area differences that exist in that same process. So, when we talked to our American parent company about the need for what became known as Life Assist, we weren't really on the same page."

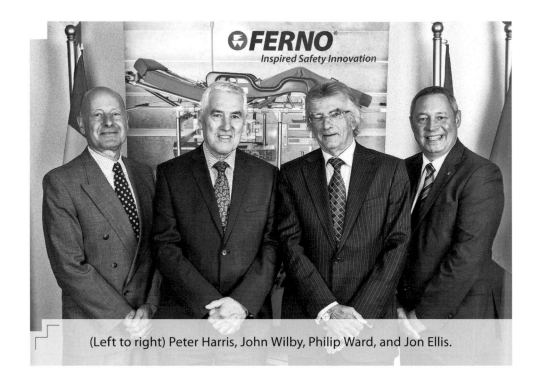

(Left to right) Peter Harris, John Wilby, Philip Ward, and Jon Ellis.

He came up with a plan to acquire a manufacturing facility nearby and made his pitch to Joe. "That's one of the benefits of the Ferno family." They listen. "So, with the approval of Wilmington, we started to design, develop and manufacture a whole new range of Lift Assist products. Fortunately for us, the market accepted it."

And Joe accepted that Philip Ward's market was in some ways different from Silvia Vancova's labor situation which was different from Simon Zerihun's opportunity which was different from Tore Larsen's customer. Thanks to his years of listening (and of collecting an outrageous number of frequent flyer miles) Joe knew the players and the unique circumstances of each. He was listening and quietly connecting the dots.

"No question. No question at all," Peter Peemans said. "That's what made the strength of Ferno International. Instead of saying 'this is what we do in the States and that's the right way to do it,' Ferno has developed products that answer the needs of a particular market abroad. We have a model for the German market. We have a model for the French market. We have a model for the UK market. And these are completely different systems. We still transport the patient. We still load and unload the patient from an ambulance, but we do it in a different way. Ferno would either modify a product or create a new product from scratch."

The humility that is part of nearly every conversation Joe or El have about their version of leadership is a personal quality. They insist on being first-named by everybody in the plant, while they, themselves, call the guy who brings them their sandwich at a restaurant "sir." But humility also has a strong and effective business purpose. Sometimes humility means you notice and acknowledge that somebody else might have a better idea, something else worth consideration. "You can get an awful lot done," El said, "if you don't care who gets the credit."

And, just as he'd hoped, Ferno moved forward with a CEO who was fully engaged and looking for new challenges.

Many air miles and meetings would lie ahead for Joe. Detours into product diversification, distractions with legal and regulatory challenges, and global competition to the core products had put a strain on the Ferno Group. For several years, Joe threw his energy toward ways to better organize and focus the organization, align the personnel, and reaffirm company's response to customers' needs.

He established low cost product sourcing and manufacturing and explored opportunities in developing markets. George Reazer, Peter Kochan and Silvia Vancova helped open Eastern Europe with Saver Manufacturing, later renamed Ferno Slovakia. In 2000, Ferno Mexico was established.

Vice President of Asia-Pacific Operations Robert DeBussey, Gary Hiles and Joe evaluated the South American market, concluding that timing and market conditions were not yet right for entry there, concentrating instead on Asia and India. In 2001, the ProFlexx Series began to roll out, and Ferno introduced the world's first composite cot. Ferno entered the veterinary market with Aqua Paws, an underwater treadmill for dogs, and Aqua Pacer, an underwater treadmill for horses.

Reflecting on those early years of his leadership, Joe said, "You never really invent anything. You just start remaking something that was done in the past," making it better, more efficient. "In early 2000, we invoked a very rigid voice of customer process to drive change throughout the entire operation." This organized listening "allows us to start to interpret things, and sometimes it's hard to connect the dots but every time you listen to a customer's comment, you think, 'Well, how can I solve that issue, that need, that challenge they have?'"

Strategy. Change. Growth. Product. But there is something else at the heart of Joe Bourgraf's vision for the company. "I think one of the unique things about emergency services or about the mortuary business is the passion of the people in it. Knowing that it could be my son, my daughter, my wife, friends or parents on that product, it just gives me that drive and passion to solve the problem."

Increasingly, Joe was convinced that future challenges would be overcome by post-modern means and original thought. There was no blueprint for Dick Ferneau and El Bourgraf to follow when *they* invented an industry, now Joe Bourgraf was poised to *re-invent* it. Computers were a given, but information technology offered up a whole new world of opportunity.

"The ways were changing," Joe said. "Gone were the days of draftsman and paper, trial and error development models, singular or narrow material selections and construction methodologies. Computers, the internet, and corresponding technology changes were evolving and dynamic, and Ferno needed to embrace the future."

He put a computer on every desk and invested in the latest design and engineering software. Safety issues were analyzed with finite element analysis (FEA) and new ideas brought to life with computer aided design (CAD). "The transition would not be easy or occur overnight," Joe said, "but over the next several years Ferno would implement and standardize on a global engineering platform, formalize structure and communication between its global companies, completely remodel the product range and brand image, all while transitioning to a more technology savvy workforce and direct market channel engagement." Remembering those years, he added, "this challenge was not easy while still managing the day-to-day business."

Then came September 11, 2001.

"Like so many in our country," Joe wrote in the company newsletter, "we will forever be indebted to all those who have given so much in responding to that week's tragic events. We grieved the loss, applauded the courage, and have been inspired by the sacrifice of so many for the good of us all. As each member of the Ferno family watched the horror unfold, and the emergency response, we should be proud of the services we provide, the real impact of our products. It makes the Ferno mission and vision statements become real."

Company attorney Bill Keating said, "As I watched the coverage of the rescue efforts, I saw the Ferno cots. Ferno emergency patient-handling products are an integral part of major rescue efforts throughout the world. Ferno makes a difference in the quality of care of the seriously injured."

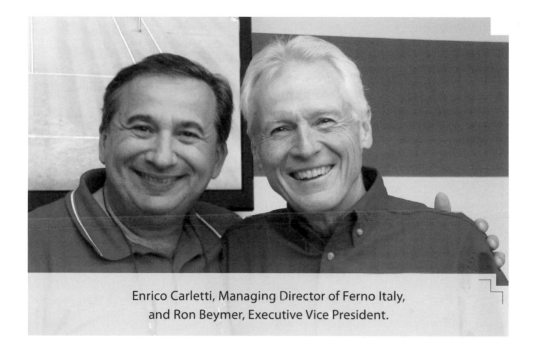

Enrico Carletti, Managing Director of Ferno Italy,
and Ron Beymer, Executive Vice President.

Anguished condolences poured in from around the world from the Ferno family, their words reflecting the fond and personal nature of the relationships El, Joe, Ron Beymer, Gary Hiles, and others had built over the years.

"I want to tell you that we share the American feelings and the sadness of these days," Enrico Carletti wrote.

"We are shocked and devastated. We pray God's guidance to you as a nation and to your country's leadership to guide your great country to full recovery soon. Tough times never last. Tough people do," said Conradie van Heerden from South Africa.

"Our sorrow is beyond what can be described in words," wrote Zernur Vardar of Istanbul. "Living in a country that has been under the threat of terrorism for many years and has suffered, we condemn any and all acts of terrorism and hope that the whole world will unite for peace."

Another Turkish friend, Melih Berk, decried the murders as an "unforgivable crime of humanity, which makes no differentiation of language, religion, or race."

Similar messages came from New Zealand, Australia, Russia, Tahiti, Germany, Israel, Mexico, the Netherlands, and the UK.

Joe immediately dispatched a donation of equipment to New York emergency workers. "Ferno employees, like the rest of the nation, are in shock and want to do anything they can to aid the victims." Subsequently the United States went to war, and Ferno did, too. A military division already was in place and Ferno was well known in Washington.

A 1999 letter came from Brigadier General Mary L. Saunders, USAF: "The overwhelming success of Operation Allied Force in Kosovo could not have happened without your responsive efforts to the demands we placed upon you." The article detailed sales to the government including cots (Models 28s, 35As and A+s, 93ESs and EXs), 175 Fasteners, 65 Scoops, and Stair Chairs.

Military purchasing agents have elephantine requirements. Quality equipment, fair pricing, and reliable delivery. Just after Sept. 11, at the request of the U.S. Department of Defense, Ferno began manufacturing a special surgical table that could be used in military transport aircraft. The table, later used by American special forces in Afghanistan, is essentially a bed on wheels with attached storage space for sophisticated medical equipment and medicine and can be used to do complex surgeries inside an aircraft and in battle zones.

In addition to the surgical tables, Ferno sold tents, chemical decontamination shelters, chemical decontamination kits, and gas masks.

When the U.S. Military Special Operations Command (SOC) went looking for a flexible and responsive company with aviation, medical, wilderness, and global experience, Ferno was ready, a proven entity. Bob Chinn, a dentist and an aviation and mechanical enthusiast who's now managing director of Ferno Aviation, seized the niche. "Bob was never much on selling to the 'big military,'" Joe said. "Special Operations was becoming the superstar among the military elite, with an integrated and multi-branch approach and a rapid strike and extraction capability." Ferno, Joe said, was nimble enough to respond to their mission specific requirements.

In addition to the Air Mobile Surgical Table, Ferno Military coordinated simple transitions in existing Ferno products, producing the Marine Trauma Bay, Strat-V Transporter, and Blackhawk Litter kit. More than thirty major or minor programs and products were manufactured to meet the new reality of terrorist threats.

"We got drawn into supporting efforts in the wars in Iraq and Afghanistan," Joe recalled. "That effort consumed a lot of engineering and manufacturing time and really shifted us out of our core market."

During the intervening years, Ferno continued to respond to the world's demands for their signature emergency equipment. The product line grew with a

35P X-frame heavy duty cot in 2002, followed by a 93P H-frame heavy duty cot in 2003. PowerFlexx, a hydraulic cot capable of lifting 700 pounds, was introduced to the market in 2005, and the company developed the 24 MAXX heavy duty mortuary cot the same year.

"Wars don't really create business for us," El said, "but people who have been there affect the civilian industry. A lot of our product innovations totally relate to our wartime experiences."

Working with military customers planted new ideas to be explored—interchangeable tools in the field, a refreshed look at the EMS environment, practical lessons on safety and efficiency. With the success of U.S. military actions and the looming presidential elections of 2008, "an air of political and global shift began," Joe said. Internal military personnel believed that Osama bin Laden was within reach, and Ferno's efforts in development and supply should start shifting back to the commercial markets they served prior to 9/11. "In 2009, we started to shift back and really focus on our core domestic and international customer base once again," Joe said. The Mondial was introduced to the European and Asian market that year, a manual cot series that continued to improve and refine the patient loading experience.

But Joe had bigger dreams. The trick would be to keep the entrepreneurial spirit that had served his father so well, while boosting Ferno from its comfortable perch as a mid-sized firm to the next rung. The management team had studied breakthrough companies that had successfully made the jump and chose the following common characteristics to model:

• Focusing resources on a few big bets.

• Systematically building character. Incorporating the best outside ideas.

• Willingness to question fundamental assumptions.

• Surrendering the sovereignty of the leader to the sovereignty of the company.

The research set the stage for gutsy new direction, driven by Joe, who had never relinquished his vision of something extraordinary, something that would represent a pivot as dramatic as the invention of the One-Man Cot. Then, along came a young engineer who kept a notebook by the side of his bed in case he thought of something brilliant in the middle of the night. And, one night, he did.

We've got some fantastic new products coming on. This company could double, triple in size fairly quickly…it's going to be exciting. It's going to be exciting for everybody here, a great future for everybody.

New Horizons

An Idea with Legs

Ferno's CEO, the second generation of leadership, once described himself as an "antsy" kid. Impatient and energetic, Joe Bourgraf wanted to get cracking on his vision for the future. The next product, the game changer, would be a stretcher that integrated the X-frame and independent legs. It could morph into a chair. It would solve problems for transporters both inside and outside the ambulance. It would be a totally independent device, self-powered without adding significant weight or bulk to the cabin of the vehicle. Capable of loading patients onto any kind of ambulance anywhere in the world, it would do all the lifting for the medics. All of it. Faster than anything else those in the EMS profession had ever seen, the iN/X would be the crucial step toward his vision for revolutionary patient transport.

First, of course, it would be safe.

"Our products," El said, "have to work in the heat of Saudi Arabia and on the ice in Sweden." Internal testing is the alpha step, supervised by the testing department's Sailesh Tangirala. "We are actually testing to how medics use the cot day-to-day in the field," he said. "Say, they roll over a curb or walk and accidentally hit a curb. Maybe they have to push through gravel or sand. Maybe the cot sits on a football field for a few hours. Or a few days. What happens to the plastics and metal on the cart? We test for the long-term life of the product."

El Bourgraf used to talk about building the Cadillac of cots, the Mercedes of stretchers. Joe's team liked to imagine the Bugatti Veyron, the most powerful and fastest production car in the world. Named in honor of a French race car driver who won the 1939 LeMans in a Bugatti, the car is exotic, sleek, and ahead of its time. The team gave considerable thought to what their new product would be called. Philip Ward loved to boast about naming his cots. "For some reason, they all had numbers. So we gave ours a name people could relate to—a lot of fun."

At first, design engineer Nick Valentino's assignment was simply to give Ferno's PowerFlexx cot a facelift. This Ferno product line was designed to reduce lifting during patient handling. Then Tim Schroeder, head of product management and Nick's mentor, wondered if the young man would like to take on something completely new instead of "just kicking the can down the road." How about figuring out a way to eliminate lifting altogether? Nick had been looking for a chance like this since he got his engineering degree in 2003 from Wright State University in Dayton.

"I wanted to do something that had meaning." He'd had false starts at small companies, where "they weren't really ready or able to invest in new products." If times got tough, they'd try to point him toward sales. He joined Ferno in August of 2007. A week later, his wife had major surgery. "Ferno said family comes first," Nick said. "I was told to go be with my wife, and they still paid me for that week—only my second week at the company."

A year and a half later, he got his big career break. Something important. Something new. "I just couldn't do it fast enough. I was very motivated." Bursting with ambition, pent up passion to make a contribution, and with a healthy dollop of loyalty, he started drawing obsessively. At his desk, at the dinner table. He kept a pad and pencil on his bedside table. "Sometimes when you're done for the day, you can stop thinking about anything else and really focus." He came up with what he calls leg geometry. "The front and back legs of the stretcher had to fold and pass through each other, powered and moving independently." A week later he was standing in the office of the vice president of operations with his design in his hands.

He sketched it out on the VP's white board. Keep going, he was told. Encouraged, he went back to the computer and booted up design software. "I was applying forces to my sketches, trying to make sure it would be practical, possible. That's another reason I was glad I was at Ferno. Top of the line software." He modeled the shape of the legs, how they would move and nest under the frame. How they would fold and pass through each other, bearing the entire weight of the patient during loading. Clearance, perspective, how this cot would be powered. It looked good on the screen. It was time for Skunkworks, which is how Dick Ferneau and El used to describe the nitty-gritty of turning their ideas into metal.

The term originated during World War II to describe a hasty campaign to build a fighter jet and morphed into industrial shorthand to describe a small group of people who worked on a project in an unconventional way. "I always thought of it as a bunch of people working together who weren't afraid to get their hands dirty," El said, reaching back into Ferno's R&D history beginning with Dielco which became the Blue Room. "Really, just guys who worked better with their hands. Some of them, like Bob Dunn, migrated there after doing other things." Dunn,

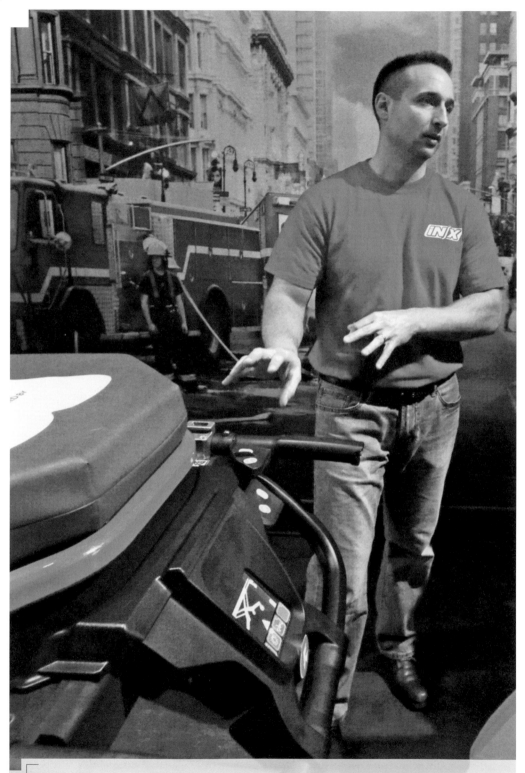

Designer Nick Valentino, a chance to be part of something special.

who joined Ferno in 1959, was promoted to foreman of the Greenfield plant in 1962, then engineering director of the Wilmington plant in 1966. "This guy had mechanical aptitude that wouldn't quit," El said. He finished out his career at Ferno in The Skunkworks.

"They'd sometimes save things they made that didn't work that might be valuable later." Ron Vance, Kenny Self—Skunkworks alumni whose names appear on several patents alongside El's—would be very familiar with the Little Red Wagon, a pet project of El's that would involve eliminating the front wheels of

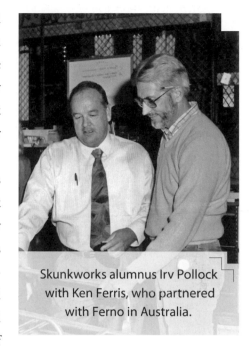

Skunkworks alumnus Irv Pollock with Ken Ferris, who partnered with Ferno in Australia.

the stretcher. "I still think it might be valuable later," El said, "maybe in the second or third generation of the iN/X."

In the 21st Century spirit of Skunkworks, Nick explained what he needed to some of the men in the shop—Scott Chambliss, Bill Benedict, Jerry Taylor. They laser cut aluminum sheets and swiped a few pieces from an existing stretcher and maybe some things they'd saved that hadn't worked before. They wrestled with the idea as well as the materials.

Soon, they had a rudimentary prototype. "A big group of people came around, a team, the ones who made the big decisions, including Joe and El," Nick said. "All I had was the frame and the legs and the supporting arm that linked the frame to the legs." No actuator, which was key. The actuator, Nick explained, "is a kind of motor, basically a cylinder driven by hydraulics." The power.

Nick stood inside the frame, held on, and used his own legs as actuators, shoving one foot forward and the other behind to raise the contraption, his beautiful/ugly contraption. "You could see it in their eyes. They got it. It clicked with everybody. They could understand what was going on." Years later, his voice still betrayed his excitement at that moment.

"That's the thing about Ferno. People here understand their products very well," Nick added. "Joe and El are great at business, but they also know design and how things work. And you have other people who have been here for a long time, who have seen what succeeds and what doesn't. The wealth of knowledge of people who had been doing this for twenty-plus years just created a perfect storm for the iN/X."

That day when Nick scissored his legs to mimic his vision of independent locomotion of four metal legs—a completely untried way to move patients—was just the beginning of an arduous and expensive process, an adventure in research and development, a test of resolve. About the same time, Bob Chinn was sharing his experiences with military tracks and mount systems. He talked to the team about the rigors of crash and blast testing and components that needed to be rigged yet lightweight and fit all types of vehicles and environments. They began to envision an Ambulance of the Future.

The team at Ferno traveled down some blind alleys, looking for different power sources. Scratched their heads over weight and cost. Mined the results of focus groups with medics and EMTs, conversations at conventions. They pushed forward. Joe estimated that it took about 250,000 man hours to get the first iN/X to the first customer. Nobody suggested that Nick turn his hand to sales, although he was brought into the larger process. Form would most emphatically follow function.

"Very quickly, I came to realize how it would affect the lives of the EMTs," he said. "That's the passion part." Talking to El, Nick said, "You always knew you were going to hear a great story and go home learning something that you would never find in a book. I have been with this project from day one, and being there for all the hills and valleys has been one terrifying but exciting ride."

The most exciting ride was yet to come. What began as a radically different stretcher became a radically different patient transport system. It would involve dozens of specialists and thousands of hours of research and meetings and arguments. It would finally walk itself over concrete highway medians and down steps and into an ambulance. It would roll injured people safely on the cobblestones of England and the deserts of Jordan. It would save the backs of thousands of EMTs all over the world.

And it would move on legs Nick Valentino sketched on a notebook next to his bed.

Earning the 001 Tag

Pegasus and the Falcon and the Harrier worked fine in the UK, where Philip sold his wares, but a global parent company with ambitions for a universal product had to consider the translation. Once, after they came up with a name they liked for the cot, it turned out to mean condom in Italian. So numbers and letters more practical, more descriptive. Despite Ferno's reputation for a willingness to customize, this product was meant to be used all over the globe. It was versatile enough to work for EMTs in America who loaded patients directly into the ambulance, as well as UK medics who used a lift gate at the back of the vehicle and for spacious German trucks and smaller Japanese vehicles.

In April of 2014, more than 30,000 emergency responders got a chance to see the new iN/X stretcher in action at a conference in Indianapolis. Built around Ferno's original X-frame but with independently functioning legs, it is the result of, as Joe said, INspiration, INnovation, INtelligence. As El said, "we like our names to mean something." And the working prototype got rave reviews:

"My first reaction?" one firefighter said. "I'm sure hoping my department will pick one up." Another said, "Awesome. Easy to load and unload." One man noticed that the independent legs would be a plus for rough terrain. "This will protect me *and* my patient." "Wow," another said. "This is the only one I've ever seen where you really don't have to lift putting it in and out of the truck. This is gonna save my back."

No wonder they liked it. Many of them had, in effect, been on the design team.

Steve Schwandner, CEO of Schwandner Creativity Center in Mason, Ohio, worked on research to "uncover and quantify customer requirements that could be translated into the product." Rajib Adhikary, CEO of KAALO, an Austin, Texas, design company, said his team worked with targeted design requirements on everything from handle grips to materials used on the finish. The Voice of the Customer (VOC) continued to produce nuggets of information that added to the Ambulance of the Future concept. As these ideas were generated, valued, and tested in the market, they were placed into the appropriate categories for the strategy team.

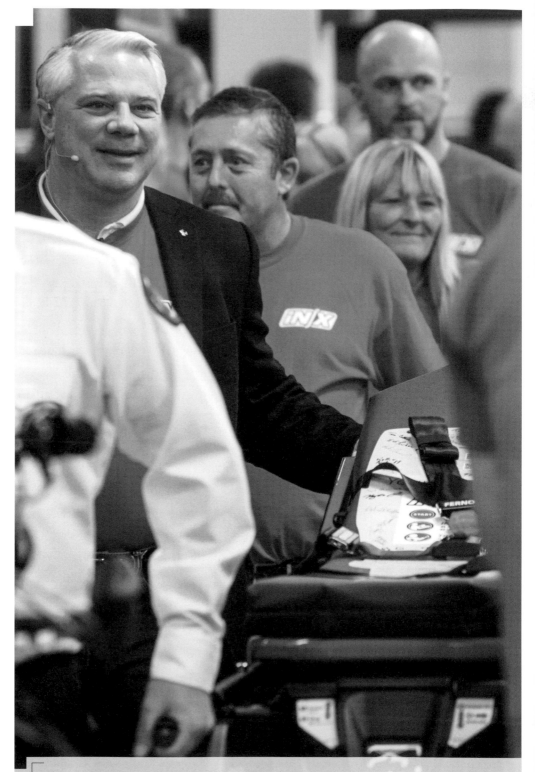

Joe and the Ferno family bring the first iN/X cot off the line, February 6, 2015.

One such effort was to list the issues and challenges faced by EMTs and EMS operators. At the top of the list was a simple word: safety. Medics were being hurt or injured on the job, as were patients during a crash or dramatic swerve. They told the Ferno researchers that medics had to be constantly moving around in the back of the ambulance, treating patients and reaching for medical supplies and devices. Descriptions, pictures, and videos were gathered, presented, and interpreted.

Ferno's product manager Jim West said, "Our goal was to extend the careers of the paramedics. We sat down with those key groups and really wiped the slate clean. What do you do in your job? How can we help you do it better?" They were looking to uncover new functions, new features, go beyond the expected, translate what they learned in creative and highly engineered ways. Before they were finished listening and engineering, they would apply for seventeen patents on the new stretcher.

In this company of open communication, enthusiasm was picking up steam. Employees had heard the buzz and they were eagerly awaiting the new stretcher's appearance in the marketplace. All the assembly and much of the fabricating would be done in Wilmington, a very big thing. Maybe late in mid-2014, it was rumored. Then it looked as if production might begin in November. In December of 2014, Joe Bourgraf stood ready to explain the delay to the troops.

More than 250 people had gathered at the Customer Experience Center. Right on cue, the CEO stepped from the wings, his wavy dark hair touched with gray. His tie, red with a thin blue and gray stripe, had a background motif with the Ferno logo.

Brisk without being brusque, commanding without arrogance, moving from baritone to bass and back again in a radio-ready, compelling voice and wearing a Madonna mic bobbing next to his face, he managed to be the only one of the speakers that day who didn't send the sound system into screeching protest. He was greeted with better than perfunctory applause. He stood in front of a blowup of the words of the retailing pioneer, J.C. Penney: "Growth is never by mere chance. It is the result of forces working together." This was the Floor Talk, a quarterly assembly of Ferno's employees who are allowed an unusually open look at the company's finances and prospects.

The CEO warmed up the crowd, announcing a $14.4 million grant from FEMA for assistance to firefighters and a new ambulance-building partnership with

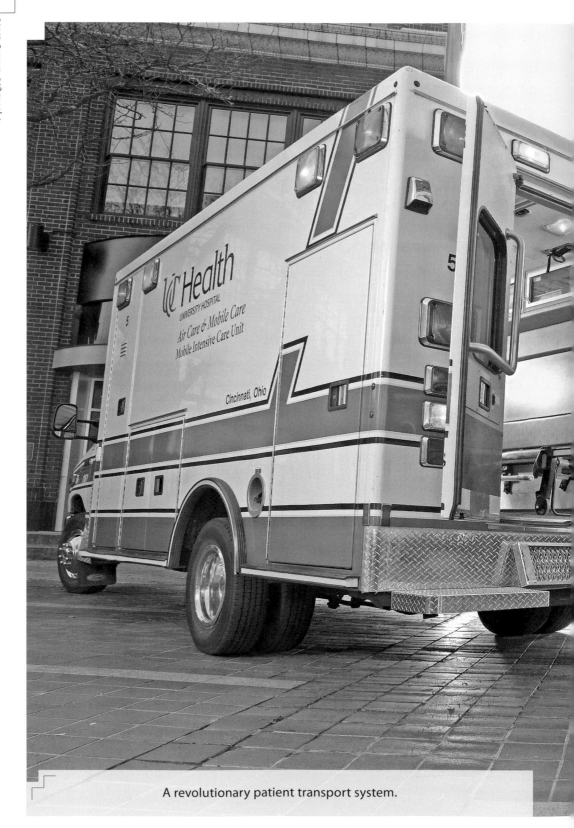

A revolutionary patient transport system.

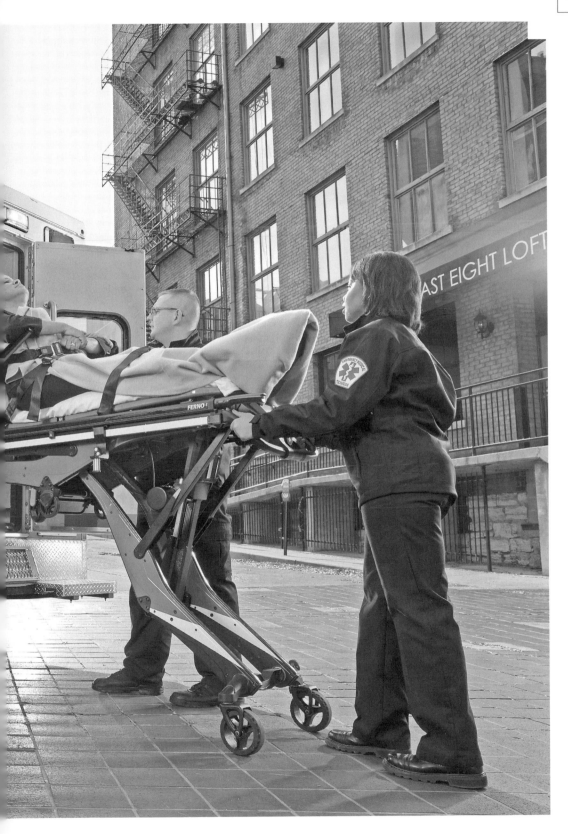

Toyota "as of thirteen seconds ago." Next, Marketing Manager Jerry Socha talked about branding and a revamped website.

The "two Tims" took turns at the mic. Tim Schroeder, now director of ambulance systems, and Tim Wells, global product manager, caught the crowd up on new products, field testing, and some of the problems that had delayed production on the iN/X—a hairline crack, an angle sensor, a problem wheel mount, an unacceptable battery charge. "It has to be *right* before we ship," Tim Wells said. People in the audience nodded. They knew what it costs to repair something. They knew what it meant to the company's reputation as well. They are Ferno-ized. Informed. They appreciate the value of the 001 Tag, which means a product is customer-ready.

The Tims flung around an alphabet soup—CEC, iN/X, IPTS—which is mysterious to no one in the audience. The Customer Experience Center (CEC) where the chairs had been set up today, has been duplicated at Ferno UK, which sent along a video of their new space. The iN/X is the stretcher of the future, and many of those in the crowd have had their hands on it. The IPTS (Integrated Patient Transport System) combines the patient/medic, environment and intelligence platforms into one solution that will add up to Joe's vision of the ultimate in intelligent design. The Ferno crew was remarkably well informed, as the quarterly Floor Talks are only part of regular communications.

As each new division and as new countries are folded into the Ferno Group, as new products are tested, these people are among the first in the world to know. Spiracle Technology, the company's emergency respiratory care products division acquired in 1995, was discussed here. When Ferno Aviation was established a year later, employees were informed. All along the way they have been included in the conversation.

Luis Gonzalez, director of international marketing, told them about a non-Ferno fire rescue equipment company which has topped more than $2 million in sales. The Ferno Military Division, which has lagged as wars in the Middle East wound down and further pinched by the government sequestration, is picking up as threats from ISIS and other terrorists escalate.

The star of this particular quarterly meeting was Paul Riordan, the popular senior vice president and chief financial officer. The crowd, already attentive, seemed to lean forward a bit as the gray-haired, bespectacled veteran started his presentation. It was the end of the company's fiscal year. October sales were a bit below budget, he said, but "we had costs under control." In November, "we exceeded plan." This was good news indeed, judging by the faces in the crowd. He shared insight about the international strength of the dollar and R&D expense.

"UK blew it out of the water this year," he confided, pointing to figures on cash collections, political consequences, competition. Jordan is buying surgical tables. The yen has been weak in Japan." He was leading up to the information the people in the audience were eagerly awaiting. They were about to see the bottom line and most of them were seasoned enough to quickly figure out their share in it. The incentive formula Ron Beymer helped put in place in 1997 had resulted in the subsequent years in checks to employees increasing their total compensation between three percent and six percent. Most years, they'd been presented with a bonus check equaling roughly two weeks' salary.

Paul hit a button and a slide of a giant Christmas tree appeared. This had to be good news. And it was. About a four percent bonus.

The management team took some questions. One long-time employee wondered why he hadn't seen many new faces in the shop. "Retirees are leaving," he said, "and not being replaced."

Joe told him Ferno is planning to drop some products from "our portfolio," and that he plans to shrink SKUs—stock keeping units—from inventory. "We will be re-balancing, and we want to make sure we do it in a responsible manner," he says. Like his father, who described dancing around the vagaries of world economics and human resources with a determination to "think creatively about keeping people, protecting jobs," Joe had a strategy of cross-training.

"Some products are going away. Skill sets have to be redeployed." The velocity of change is increasing. Outside forces are changing. Three topics were on Joe's mind as he inched his new stretcher toward the marketplace: the Affordable Care Act, safety regulations, and accreditation and protocols defined by the American College of Emergency Physicians (ACEP). All of these elements are evolving. All of them have impact on Ferno products. And the evolution is taking place at different rates in different states, indeed in different counties, just as his father had predicted more than two decades earlier.

In closing remarks, Joe said, "We have to think differently, adapt to the change we have to make. We have to communicate inside and outside." Hewing to the strategy prompted by the "breakthrough" focus on a few big bets, Ferno had already sold its Ille divisions. The iN/X is a very, very big bet with a price tag for development which might be as high as in the double digit millions.

Echoing Joe's simple test for market viability, his managing director in the Middle East, Simon Zerihun, predicted enormous opportunity in his part of the world. "Dubai has become the leader in the EMS area, and everybody in the region is following Dubai. Ferno is well known there," he said, "dominant. We have won the attention of everybody. So, to really follow up with new ideas and new technologies, believe me, we can be dominant, still, in that area."

Paul Riordan, reflecting on his years with Ferno, said, "We've got some fantastic new products coming on. This company could double, triple in size fairly quickly. And there's part of me that wishes I was younger so I could participate in that ride because I think it's going to be exciting. It's going to be exciting for everybody here, a great future for everybody. It's going to be neat to look back twenty years from now and see how much growth there was in the company and just see if we can get in all 196 countries. I hope we do by then. I think we will."

At the end of the meeting, bonus checks—the revenue sharing that is tangible evidence of each employee's part in the company's success and incentive for the future—were handed out. As executives put envelopes in the hands of their Ferno family members, they greeted and thanked each one—by name.

Back to the Future

The cavernous room where Ferno now holds its Floor Talks has history. When the building was part of the Air Force Base, the space was used by the CIA as a data center. The floor was raised to accommodate the tangle of connectors they needed when computers were the size of Volkswagens and nothing was wireless. After El Bourgraf and his crew moved in, it was the perfect size for rows of women and men at humming sewing machines, cutting and stitching mattresses and covers for cots.

When the scissoring and sewing was outsourced, it was just a big empty room again, a waste of space right at the heart of the front wing of the building, begging for something grand. After a year and a million dollars, it came to be very grand indeed. And even El, who dragged his heels at the idea and the expense, was won over by the project—the Customer Experience Center.

Beginning about 2008, Joe started making it part of his routine to visit the room. He drew Larry Newberry into his project. Then he began talking to a building contractor. "I wanted the room to be something special," Joe said. "I didn't want it to be just a showroom. I wanted to engage all their senses." And he wanted it to be useful and modern and, well, he just expected he could wring a lot out of his company's investment in this room.

The entrance is marked by a theatrical three-dimensional scene of an ambulance plowing through a stone wall, complete with scattered bricks and flashing lights. The windshield is an oversized video monitor, flashing the daily message. This is a dramatic business.

"We never did a single drawing," Joe said. "It was a series of conversations." And observations. Joe had the dropped ceiling removed and added a hand-painted sky. A faux road cuts through the room with a real manhole cover and a red fire hydrant. The authenticity and fierce attention to detail would not surprise anybody who knows Joe or who has visited his mother and father's basement recreation of an open air produce market.

Enormous murals of city scenes around the world are carefully lighted with tracks that can mimic day or night atmosphere. Electrical outlets and doors are

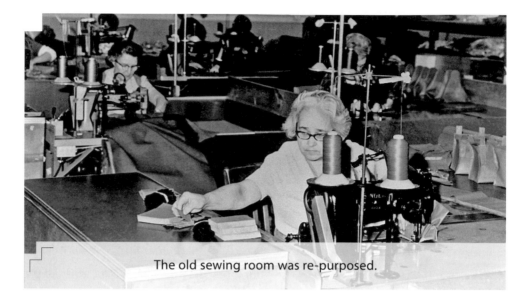

The old sewing room was re-purposed.

hand painted to blend and disappear. An "auto dealership" door allows a vehicle, say, an ambulance, to be driven in if needed. The industrial look of the entrance is carefully masked by an overlay of a firehouse door. The shell of an ambulance is always there, on a hydraulic base, easily moved for product demonstrations or video shoots of everything from the latest beriatric equipment for very large people to neonatal equipment for very tiny ones.

"We use the room every day," Joe said with satisfaction, "for webcasts, podcasts, gatherings, interviews." The sound system is state-of-the-art but the mood and tone depends on where the eye lands.

Visitors on the way to the room pass by The Wall. Stretching about fifty feet down a corridor, the floor-to-ceiling multi-media experience is layered in three topics—people, products, industry—and begins in 1854. The string of photos and information begins with a picture of the two-pole stretcher, or litter, and segues to wheeled litters, which emerged during the Crimean War. It is a typically generous homage to pioneers who preceded those at Ferno. The first person identified by name is Joseph Bomgardner, who in 1910 introduced the four-wheel swivel stretcher, later refining it by adding an adjustable backrest and a drop foot, making it a chair cot.

Then comes William Klever, who invented the all aluminum cot and gave Dick Ferneau his first job in the mortuary business, followed by Burt Weil, then Dick Ferneau and, finally, the Bourgrafs. The timeline layered below the people details the progression of mortuary and emergency products, most notably the One-Man

Cot, forerunner of all modern ambulance cots invented by Burt Weil, engineered by Dick Ferneau and marketed by El Bourgraf, and the Model 30, the first X-frame multi-level cot and harbinger of the iN/X.

Industry changes and global growth are traced at about knee level, repeating the "simple test," the guiding marketing direction of this company. "As a society becomes more prosperous and increases the quality of life, it becomes more focused on the care of the sick and injured, taking better care of its people."

When customers arrive at 70 Weil Way, they receive a Ferno VIP bag with a package of chocolate buckeyes paying homage to the state tree, the buckeye tree. If they are international customers, they will see their own flag flying, alongside the U.S. flag and the ISO certification flag. Their name will be on a sign in the lobby. Then, they will be led to the CEC through passages with bright lettering: iNnovation, iNspired, iNtelligence. And on the return trip, they walk beneath the question, "Are you iN?"

Joe's genius has been to push this historic company to grasp every modern tool, every computer-assisted opportunity available to it without squandering its most valuable asset—its people. He asked—no, insisted—that Ferno talent spread throughout the world come together face-to-face in cramped meeting rooms, dragging them out of their comfort zones to argue and discuss new ideas, to hash out problems amid stacks of flip charts, post-it notes, and piles of books.

Ron Beymer suggested that Joe consider adding an outside adviser to the mix. He had a name—Dr. Rajan Kamath. Joe consulted John Goering from the Goering Center at UC, where El had both personal and professional ties. John Goering was a fraternity brother of El's, and El had been a founding member in support of his friend. The Goering Center became one of the leading programs in the country in preparing the next generation of family business owners to manage the family firm.

With a strong endorsement of the Ferno leadership team, its global managing directors and the Goering Center's enthusiastic support, Joe concluded that the timing was right to initiate a Strategic Planning Team led by Dr. Kamath, who teaches at both UC's Lindner Business School and at Notre Dame and is highly regarded for his research into strategic positioning, technology management, breakthroughs by design, and change by design. "Finding a doctoral degreed individual, well published and having worked with well-known brands worldwide in our own backyard was too good an opportunity to pass up," Joe said.

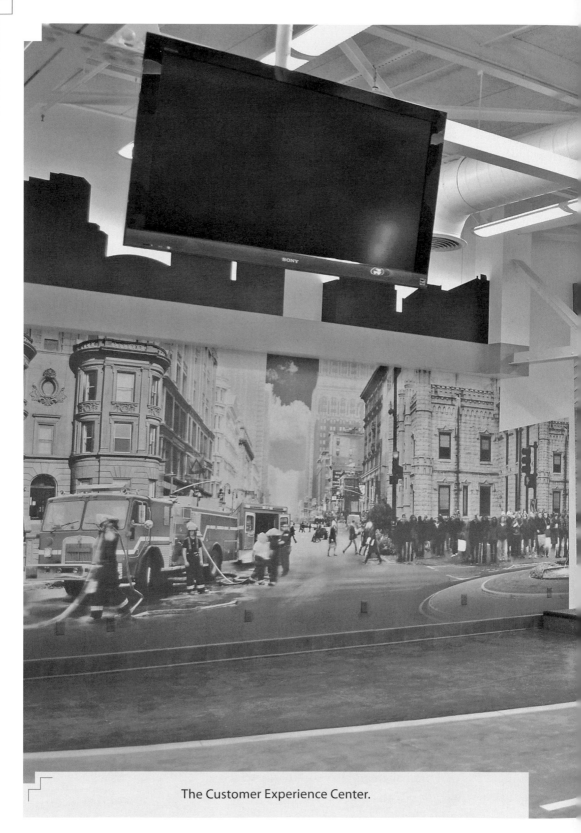

The Customer Experience Center.

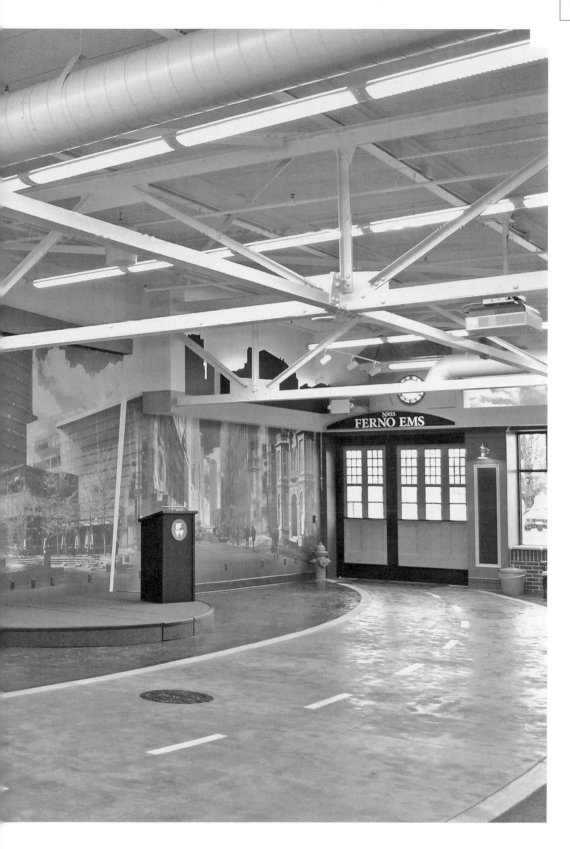

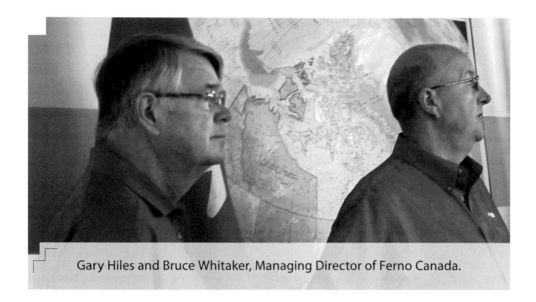

Gary Hiles and Bruce Whitaker, Managing Director of Ferno Canada.

The original Strategic Planning Team, led by Dr. Kamath, began working in 2009 and included El-B, Joe, Gary Hiles, Ron Beymer, Paul Riordan, Tim Schroeder and Bob Chinn, as well as Bruce Whitaker, Jon Ellis, and Scott West, managing directors from Canada, UK, and Australia.

Scott West, according to Jon, "always got the short straw, having to travel the most miles to the meetings, which were mostly held in the USA." And thanks to the time zone, "he was always the one on the conference calls late at night." Over the next twenty-four months, that team would meet quarterly, leading to a genuinely global design team. "A component was made in Australia," Jon said. "Another made in Slovakia, and the final product designed in the USA. This was a shift from totally relying on Wilmington and utilized Ferno Group resources to the maximum."

With each meeting, Joe said, the synergy of the group gained momentum. "You could feel innovation about to happen." They plunged into new books, strategic papers, and studied other business successes. "It was a free flow of ideas, an exchange between a group of leaders within Ferno that had the best interest of the customers and the company as their focus," Joe remembered. He often uses the telephone operator skit by the comedian, Lily Tomlin, to describe his role. "Hold on," he would say, "let me connect you." And that he did. Ideas, concepts, principles, and resourceful thinking, all brought about a series of breakthroughs that when properly aligned would bring about an Ambulance of the Future, a strategy Ferno continues to pursue today.

They completed their assignment in three years, then Ron Beymer started making noises about his own plans to head south, where he has a place in Destin, Florida. He agreed to stay for a while, implementing the findings of the group, working with managing directors around the world to set goals and, more important, to devise specific projects to get to the goals.

Next, Joe wanted a 20/20 plan. He pulled in Ron, Paul Riordan, and Raj. "The great thing about Joe—and El, too," Ron said, "is that they are looking at the company's long-term growth. Some

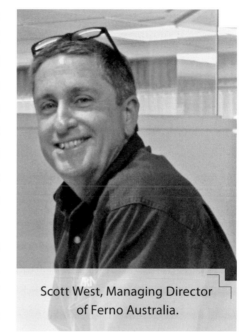

Scott West, Managing Director of Ferno Australia.

years, the bottom line might not look as good because the company has been spending money on R&D, on making that next step forward." Joe, with help from Ron Beymer and Dr. Kamath, mapped out an ambitious goal for the last half of the decade. By the year 2020, they forecast revenues of $500 million, forty percent of that from new products and services. They worked on a succession plan for all Ferno's key positions.

The marketing and sales team, led by Jerry Socha, continued to listen to customers, gaining insight, testing concepts and ideas. "Each effort and activity produced nuggets of information that were coming together to build the Ambulance of the Future," Joe said. As the customer and safety information was being researched and absorbed, Joe reached out for an expert in EMS safety to join the team, finding and hiring Jim Love who had been director of safety for one of the largest services in the United States.

No doubt about it, Joe Bourgraf is a big-picture guy. Some in the Ferno family call him a visionary. He is also the rare executive who, like his father, is also attentive to detail. El Bourgraf worked with the architect who designed the movie set rendition of Findlay Market in his basement, right down to a curb eroded by a leaky, authentic hydrant. Like his mother, Joe embraces his history. He presides over a multi-million-dollar EMS company which owes its start to the mortuary business.

So, amid the webcast-ready equipment and the hydraulic ambulance shell and the murals of busy foreign cities is another scene, at one end of the room on a back wall—a cemetery, peaceful and deserted, with a single Joshua Tree as sentry, a tree whose branches symbolize a process of coming to be, a dynamic of turning from the past, in order to achieve a new orientation.

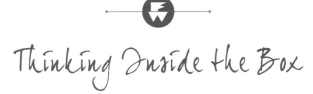

Thinking Inside the Box

El Bourgraf held the future of Ferno in his hand. He fiddled with his cell phone until he found the image he sought—an amateur video of a 9-year-old boy loading his six-foot-six, 260-pound father into an ambulance. Using the iN/X stretcher's power instead of his own back or muscle, the kid easily slides his dad into the ambulance. Actually, the cot appears to crawl into the ambulance. The boy grins, and his father gives him a high five. El laughed delightedly. "This will totally change the industry. It will be an engineer's nightmare to try to compete with this. We have raised the bar. This is pure Joe," he said, giving his own son an enthusiastic verbal thumbs up. "Joe's understanding of technology played a large part in taking the company to another level."

When Joe asked his management team to work with him on what came to be called the Integrated Patient Transport System (IPTS), he already knew that the iN/X would be just the first chapter of the story. He was sitting, literally, on the next chapter. The seed was sown during a break in the hallway at a Strategy Team meeting. "Hey, Joe," one of the managing directors said, "do you remember that sketch, the one with a chair hanging from the ceiling on a track?"

The following Monday, Joe was back in his office digging through files to discover "that sketch." He started investigating the array of ergonomic chairs available around the world. He bought several of them, mostly designed for office use, and teetered on them and pushed and pulled, imagining a medic trying to work on a patient, trying to grab a piece of equipment while the ambulance bounced and shifted.

One Sunday, Joe demonstrated one of his best seating candidates to his friend Dr. Jim Augustine, an emergency physician with an impressive array of teaching titles, as well as thirty years' service in emergency medicine. Augustine has worked on many of the national committees and boards that have shaped modern EMS and carries fireman turnout gear in the back of his car—just in case.

Joe and Jim paced off a space in Joe's garage corresponding roughly to the interior of an ambulance. They tried out Joe's favorite chair—a $1,200 Scandinavian kneeling chair with a back rest and wooden runners. They liked the chair's range of motion and its versatility. Medics come in all shapes and sizes, so they also considered adjustments they'd need to make.

They spent a whole day with "What happens if...?" scenarios. The size of patients. The size of the emergency. The procedures. Now that Joe had what he believed was the perfect patient platform in the iN/X, he was bent on finding the perfect platform for the medic, one that would let him move from the head-to-toe of the patient, able to reach any medication or tool he needed, still seated and still safe. Joe had found a chair he liked. Now he needed a way to keep the medic strapped in safely but still able to move around the patient. He needed to find the right restraints for his medic chair, plus mobility rails and tracks.

"Nothing is original," Joe said. "Not really. We started looking at other environments. NASA. NASCAR." Bob Chinn continued to remind the team of the military approach to "develop and define the interface, allowing me to meet the flexibility, modularity, and interchangeability that the military required to quickly adapt to each mission." Bob showed them Power Point demonstrations of a Cougar program, where a row of three seats could fold down to provide a litter for wounded soldiers. Thinking about the magic combination of speed and safety amid massive jolts, the team started talking about roller coasters. Somebody Googled roller coaster manufacturers and up popped a Thrill Ride Industry Convention in Las Vegas coming up in a few days. Joe booked a flight.

By the time he returned to Wilmington, he had spoken to not only every major builder of metal coasters, but to the manufacturer in Pennsylvania who made the seats for everybody in the industry. And just like El, who in Gary Hiles estimation learned from "the guy sitting next to him on a plane," Joe struck up a conversation in the Salt Lake City Airport and learned that Dr. Ned Hansen, one of the industry's outstanding engineers, was starting his own company.

Joe made a call two weeks later. "We are not in the business of manufacturing ambulances, but I need to figure out how to restrain a medic in a chair."

"I think I can work on that," said Dr. Hansen, who holds a doctorate degree in mechanical engineering and before he started his consulting business was chief engineer for one of the most innovative ride manufacturers in the world. "Ned brought knowledge and engineering capacity, not to mention the fact that his designs had to accommodate ninety-five percent of mankind. Kids, adults, pear shapes." The team came up with the skeleton of a chair and used crash dummies to test it against the Federal Motor Vehicle Safety Standards (FMVSS).

Joe paired Ned up with Jim Love, now program manager for Ferno's ACETECH, another piece of the puzzle, another chapter in the IPTS story. At their first Ambulance Chair Team meeting, Ned and Jim sat in a suite at the Little America Hotel in downtown Salt Lake City. Using a couch, coffee table, and chair to simulate what goes on in the back of an ambulance, modeling what medics do, talking about restraints, lap bars and body ergonomics, they were off and running to design a safe seating environment.

Armed with a Power Point on the issues, the topic of safety in the ambulance and a video clip of the Ambulance of the Future animation, Joe visited medical directors, large services, individual medics, insurance underwriters, government regulatory agencies, and anybody else who would listen. One of those chance encounters was with Matt Crossman, at the time Director of Operations for Medive in Nova Scotia. "Have you bumped into that Irish chap who is presenting that new control system for the back of the ambulance?" he asked Joe.

By 2010, Joe had established ACETECH, which brought data and electronic communication and control into the equation. ACETECH would warn the medic when the ambulance was about to make a turn with a vibration on the seat under his thighs. It would automatically put the engine on idle at the scene of an accident. The IPTS team began figuring out new ways for the medic to communicate with the driver, with his dispatcher, with the hospital, with other medical devices, with the outside world.

The cot, the chair, the communications. One more important chapter was yet to be written—the box. "If you look at the back of an ambulance, you realize that it hasn't changed in thirty years. It's still a metal box with a bunch of cabinets," Joe said. "What if you took out all the cabinets and opened up the space?" Drawing upon Ferno's experience with the military, the team began to think about components that could be secured to docking stations on the sides of the box, kits that contained specific tools needed for the medical emergency ahead. Everything they needed and nothing they didn't. They might look like suitcases, maybe with handles so they could be pulled from the wall of the ambulance and into the accident scene.

Cabinets? Creative storage? They went to Fort Wayne, Indiana, RV Center of planet Earth, the perfect place to look for solutions that would work in any box around the world. This was also a place that specialized in using every square inch of compartment space. It was more breakthrough thinking by a team looking for creative and efficient ways to mount

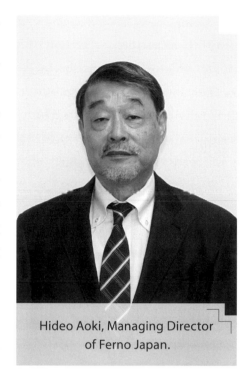

Hideo Aoki, Managing Director of Ferno Japan.

wiring, light fixtures, cameras, USB data ports, and power stations. Chris Way, vice president of global marketing who came to Ferno in 2013, called it a "soft wall system." It allows any customer to customize the ambulance to their own singular use. "Whether they're usually making emergency runs or if they need ALS (Advanced Life Support) capabilities, they can customize the vehicle."

New guidelines for ambulance compartments are being developed by the Department of Homeland Security (DHS) and the National Institute for Occupational Safety and Health (NIOSH) to address crash worthiness, worker safety and performance, and patient safety. These will include seat and restraints, stretcher and patient restraints, compartment layout and work flow, storage, ingress and egress, lighting, workspace and communications. Joe intends that Ferno's system will meet or exceed anything global regulations can throw at the EMS industry.

Jon Ellis, Ferno UK's managing director and part of Joe's strategic planning team, has been working with end users and vehicle builders there, "engaging with customers, showing them what's coming through, sowing the seeds. Nothing more exciting than having innovation coming through." He knows, "It's gonna take a transformation in thinking because of vehicle modifications and other things necessary to implement it."

Alain Mampuya, managing director of VanDePutte Medical, Ferno's distribution partner in Belgium, the Netherlands, and Luxembourg, suggested, "It will link the ambulance business much more into the whole chain of events," winning more time and better outcomes for the patient.

Ferno sponsored a 2020 Vision series in 2013 to bring together industry experts. Matt Zavadsky of Medstar Mobile Healthcare in Dallas told the audience, "We are not just the pre-hospital, not the out-of-hospital, not the after-hospital. We are part of the health system." Joe's friend, Dr. Jim Augustine challenged listeners to "imagine in 2020 that we don't have to use the hospital as the center of the healthcare system. Imagine if we could just say wherever they choose to be is the center of the healthcare system."

In February of 2015, the first iN/X was assembled for delivery. It took fifteen hours. Exuberant employees, including the CEO, dressed in jeans and red t-shirts to watch the iN/X roll down a red carpet. The unstuffy CFO Paul Riordan donned gigantic flashing green sunglasses. El's pre-recorded video message for the launch, also exuberant, ended with, "Go for it!"

Joe reminded the crowd of about 350 that "the patient is at the center of everything we do" and cut a red ribbon, sending the iN/X on its way to the Brooklyn Heights Fire Department, outside of Cleveland. Afterward, he recounted the history of the industry and Ferno's place in it, then invited the crowd to celebrate with drinks and food including red and white frosted cupcakes baked by Sandy Reiley in Quality Control. No matter its size and place in the world, this is still a family company.

"My vision for the business," El said, "concentrated on the handling of the patient and easing the strain on the EMT. Joe took Ferno from that level of concern to the next level, protecting them by changing and controlling their environment and equipment." Ferno continues to advance the ACETECH electronic control system, the iN/X Patient Transport and Loading System, iN/Traxx and SafeMount Environment Platform and the iN/Medic Chair.

As Ferno's 2020 Vision project moved toward completion, or, better still, toward the waiting customers, it was a textbook case of what El often refers to as evolution—not turning points, certainly not ah-ha moments. Successes and delays, technical challenges, regulatory restraints, protocol changes, partnerships. People like El and Dick, Joe and Ned, Ron and Raj, putting their heads together with a common purpose. George Reazer, hired in 1984 as an engineer and eventually named vice president of manufacturing, said of Ferno, "A little bit happens very often."

"The challenges, though, are blending the various things and knowing whether it's a dead end street or we just have to work harder or look at it differently. Once you have the idea," Joe Bourgraf said, "you keep poking at it, refining it, making it better." Or open up the view to an outsider. Knowing when to, as Ron Beymer's plan said, "incorporate the best outside ideas."

Ferno's inside ideas has led to a company that has never lost its way, with the enduring message that everybody matters. Every foot forward since 1955 has been driven by the character and integrity and values of its founders. People who worked or now work at Ferno have been helped when they needed it and educated when they desired it, beyond the expected and exceeding the requirements. Barriers are removed between the people who made the product and those who sell it and those who count the money. Employees are still encouraged to speak up, and they trust management enough to do so. They are reminded that their work has crucial human consequence.

"We're a whole lot more than a stretcher company," Joe would say.

And they always will be.

Epilogue

As El Bourgraf moves through his 80s, he's kept his thick hair, his self-deprecating humor, and his quick mind. He and Elaine ("Kunk") continue to throw open the doors of their homes in Cincinnati and Naples to assorted family and international friends. And the man who spent a lifetime stubbornly heaping credit on others begins to think about what he has accomplished, remembering how it had happened, and why.

If he had to guess when he first knew what he wanted out of life, he thinks it might have been when he organized a carnival at his grade school in Terrace Park, Ohio. It had all the elements: exciting, fun, complicated, colorful, and *useful*. And, he was in charge.

At the time, a loaf of bread cost about eight cents, so a nickel a ride seemed like good pricing strategy, about as far as he could push it. Finding jobs for everyone who wanted to help, he counted the proceeds at the end of the day and came up with $15 to give to the Red Cross. "I was an entrepreneur long before I knew the meaning of the word. I was living it." Elated but unsatisfied, he began thinking about next year, how he could do it better.

Like the entrepreneur he so admired, Carl Lindner, who used to hand out gold flag cufflinks engraved with the words "Only in America," El believes he owes much to the lucky accident of being born in this country. Even when mired in a regulatory or legal morass, he found solace that it was taking place in the "best place to live and raise a family." Moreover, he understood the American pioneer spirit, taking on risk to get where you wanted to be. He would tell his grandchildren, "If you determine your destination, it's easier to plan the route. I never thought I would fail. I knew it wouldn't be smooth, but I knew I would always find a way."

Although he often says that he owes much to the University of Cincinnati, which he's backed up with generous donations, he has no qualms about having plotted his own course. The work/study program there "helped me figure out what I didn't want to do," he often explains, adding that after graduation, "I never felt that I was going to work." It was "just another day of doing what I like."

His undergraduate internship with a canny dress salesman was a lesson in the art of listening to the customer. The introductory course was taught to him by

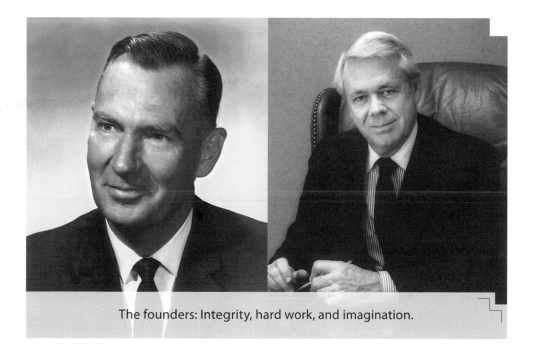

The founders: Integrity, hard work, and imagination.

his father, a casket salesman. And El passed the lesson on to his own sons. Right around the time of the launch of the iN/X, one of the most important events in his career, Joe learned that a customer was disgruntled by the prospect of late delivery of a stretcher. So, after a full work day, the young CEO loaded one in his SUV and delivered it personally late that night during a snowstorm to a fire department three hours away.

An inventor with his name attached to fourteen patents, El was, too, a businessman able to grasp the commercial possibilities of his creations. Astonishingly, he was able to manufacture them and amass success in an atmosphere of civility and respect, a tough merchant with a generous heart and a fierce competitor with character and decency. He never took anything that did not belong to him, including credit. After Dick Ferneau bowed out of the partnership, El drove the company forward without benefit of a board of directors or an old boy network of money and power.

Humble and gifted, he may believe that the traits that brought him success are common to all of us. Maybe Mickey Mantle thought if everybody really concentrated and practiced long enough, they'd be able to knock the hide off a baseball. "If I can do it, anybody can," El often said. He'd saunter through the plant with a word here and there, repeating cautionary tales to sales reps at conventions,

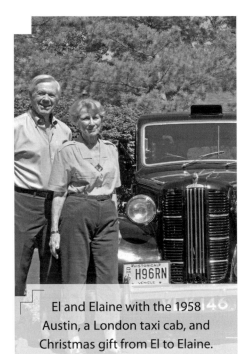

El and Elaine with the 1958
Austin, a London taxi cab, and
Christmas gift from El to Elaine.

advising executives in conference rooms from Wilmington to England to Germany to Japan. He insists he learned more than he taught.

"I never really felt I was good at anything, but I always thought I could find somebody who could do it." Dick, Bernie, Les, Rolf, Tore, Gary, Ron, Joe. He had the strength of character, the charisma, and the confidence to surround himself with talent and convince them to follow his lead. One of his international friends sorted through the English he knew, struggling to define Elroy Bourgraf, finally pronouncing him *"immediately trustable."*

Immediately trustable too, because El was careful to never put a communication out that wasn't meticulously and thoughtfully penned. A leader for over a half-century, El always felt passionate about the importance of the written word, as both a precursor to a face-to-face conversation and a powerful negotiating tactic. Notes and letters to his partner, his sons, his department managers; bulletins, newsletters, and notes to a fellow in the shop—a veritable archive exists of El's thoughts and advice on subjects as wide-ranging as behavior, mechanics, ethics, systems, and interpersonal relationships. Often times, El found a well thought-out note helped smooth over a difficult conversation and minimized the risk of an emotionally charged reaction, allowing the recipient to better absorb the message. Rebellious teens, disgruntled suppliers, employees who needed a pat on the back—or a kick in the pants—El held his tongue and picked up a pen.

"If you say something, your tone of voice might imply something you don't mean, especially if the subject is contentious. If you take the time to write it down, you can soften or rephrase. I always felt like it kept me from putting my foot in my mouth. And I would really work on it, making sure it said what I really meant."

His sincere belief was, and still is, that the spoken word had wings and could be easily misinterpreted and forgotten, but the written word could be read and reread, mulled over and absorbed in a way the spoken word could not. Looking back, he recognizes the effectiveness of this approach, his signature approach, both literally and figuratively.

"I ordered a batch of stationery fifteen years ago and still have most of it," he laughs. Reflecting on a life of successful personal and professional give-and-take, he says carefully chosen written words "have been one of my prime negotiating tools."

President of his high school class during his junior year, student body president when he was a senior, president of his fraternity when he was in college, "I still keep in touch with people from my high school. Those who are still alive." El concedes, "Maybe I was kind of a leader."

Kind of? He located talent, from Wilmington, Ohio, and Bradford, England, and Oslo, Norway, and fused them together in common purpose.

When he began peddling mortuary equipment, there was not much to sell. Some stretchers, a few of them on wheels. Then, there was lift. And life. The elevating stretcher changed the way the world carried its sick and wounded. It came out of El's partnership with Dick Ferneau and his work ethic and his charismatic leadership. The most obvious legacy is to the industry he shaped. But the most indelible one is to family, both the Ferno family and his Bourgraf kin. The two families, to him, are inextricably linked. He's bequeathed to them not rows of numbers and stretchers and cots, but an authentic model of character.

At a family meeting in 2015, he told his children, "The twilight of life should be the time to appraise life experiences, pursue and maintain principles and values that have been the foundation of what success the Lord has granted." He named the virtues he most admired as "sincerity, honesty, perseverance, unselfishness, humility and, most important, hard work, pledging to "set an example and counsel when asked." Proud of their accomplishments, he hoped they'd "grow proudly in self-esteem, confidence, and mutual respect with strong moral value."

El followed thoughtfully the progress of the new patient transport system *imagineered* by his eldest son. He poked at it with questions along the way—"Is it too high? Too heavy? Too expensive?" He stalked the Internet looking for pretenders and poachers. The family company, after nearly sixty years, continues to be driven by innovation, setting the agenda for an industry. It's clear that the seeds El planted for this new generation have taken root.

When the first iN/X was assembled in Wilmington and sent on its way to a fire department in an Ohio village near Cleveland, El applauded from his electronic vantage point in Florida. Confident of the daily leadership, the lessons learned, and the workmanship, he remains the chairman of the enterprise, looking forward, he says, to what Ferno's engineers will do in 2020 and beyond.

"One of the things on my life bucket list was to transition the Ferno team to the next generation. Under Joe's leadership, the second generation has arrived, and I take great pride in this," El says.

And as he had so many years before when he first confronted his destiny, El begins to think of next year, and how Joe and his team could do it better.

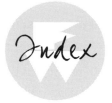

Index

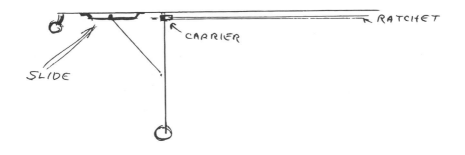

RATCHET

CARRIER

SLIDE

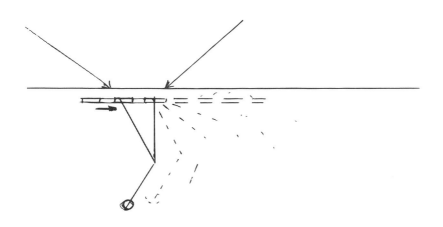

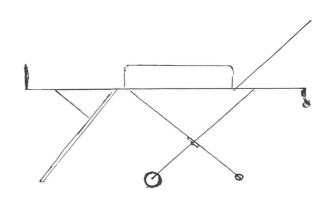